D0415310

The Sensational Baby Sleep Plan

www.rbooks.co.uk

The Sensational Baby Sleep Plan

Alison Scott-Wright

BANTAM PRESS

LONDON · TORONTO · SYDNEY · AUCKLAND · JOHANNESBURG

TRANSWORLD PUBLISHERS
61–63 Uxbridge Road, London W5 5SA
A Random House Group Company
www.rbooks.co.uk

First published in Great Britain
in 2010 by Bantam Press
an imprint of Transworld Publishers

Copyright © Alison Scott-Wright 2010

Alison Scott-Wright has asserted her right under the Copyright, Designs
and Patents Act 1988 to be identified as the author of this work.

The information in this book reflects the author's own opinions and methods, but is not
intended as a substitute for advice from a qualified medical practitioner. Always consult a
qualified medical practitioner before starting, changing or stopping any medical treatment.
So far as the author is aware, the information given is correct and up to date as at date of
publication. Practice, laws and regulations all change, and the reader should obtain up-to-
date professional advice on any such issues. The author and publishers disclaim, as far as
the law allows, any liability arising directly or indirectly from the use, or misuse, of the
information contained in this book.

A CIP catalogue record for this book
is available from the British Library.

ISBN 9780593062814

This book is sold subject to the condition that it shall not,
by way of trade or otherwise, be lent, resold, hired out,
or otherwise circulated without the publisher's prior
consent in any form of binding or cover other than that
in which it is published and without a similar condition,
including this condition, being imposed on the
subsequent purchaser.

Addresses for Random House Group Ltd companies outside the UK
can be found at: www.randomhouse.co.uk
The Random House Group Ltd Reg. No. 954009

The Random House Group Limited supports The Forest Stewardship
Council (FSC), the leading international forest-certification organization. All our
titles that are printed on Greenpeace-approved FSC-certified paper carry the FSC logo.
Our paper procurement policy can be found at www.rbooks.co.uk/environment

Typeset in 11.5/15pt Berkeley Book
by Falcon Oast Graphic Art Ltd.

Printed and bound in Great Britain
by CPI Mackays, Chatham, ME5 8TD

2 4 6 8 10 9 7 5 3 1

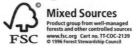

Mixed Sources
Product group from well-managed
forests and other controlled sources
www.fsc.org Cert no. TT-COC-2139
© 1996 Forest Stewardship Council
FSC

This book is dedicated to my mother, Barbara Wright, without whom it would never have been written and who has finally, after forty-five years, realized that 'the baby stage' is the easy bit!

With three daughters, six grandchildren and three great-grandchildren, she has learned not to judge but just to accept and offer her unconditional support to help deal with the many difficult challenges of family life.

Through every twist and turn, every high and low, and every page of this book, she has been there for me.

Thanks, Mum. You are my rock and I love you.

Contents

Foreword

It is with great pleasure that I write the foreword for *The Sensational Baby Sleep Plan*. I have known Alison professionally for many years, and am impressed by her practical and pragmatic approach. She has tremendous and rather valuable experience with babies who have feeding difficulties, reflux, and sleep problems, and her practical and clinical skills are helpful to many families and young children.

This book offers easy-to-follow, practical guidance and valuable advice to all families with babies, especially those who are distressed and 'colicky'. I have looked after children and babies with such problems for the last fifteen years, and during this time I have sadly seen babies who experience varying episodes of pain, distress, and/or feeding difficulties. The majority of babies with 'colic' often look well and may even be smiling whilst in the doctor's waiting room; in this situation, they can pass a normal clinical examination and often gain weight in a satisfactory manner, especially during the early stages. It is only possible for most health professionals to correctly understand the extent of the problem that both babies and parents experience if they monitor the progress of the baby over a number of hours or days, and this is what Alison specializes in.

Alison's experience with infants and babies is presented with great clarity within this book, along with some valuable hints and practical tips which, in my opinion, would be extremely useful for all parents and carers of young babies.

Over the years, working alongside Alison has proved to be productive and rewarding to both parents and their babies. I hope that this book will contribute further to the awareness of parents and health professionals in the management of babies with 'colic', reflux and feeding difficulties.

Dr Muftah Eltumi PhD, FRCP, FRCPCH
Consultant paediatric gastroenterologist
The Portland Hospital for Women and Children

1

Sleep Matters

I have put together this straightforward, easy-to-follow plan based on my years of experience working with the families of newborns. It involves neither demand feeding nor a strictly regimented routine, but is a realistic plan that strikes a happy medium between the baby's needs and the flexibility required in a busy family. The plan helps parents in today's pressurized society to relax into parenthood with confidence and a growing understanding of all it entails.

I am fully aware that the existing government guidelines on feeding and babycare are set out to promote your baby's health and wellbeing, but they are not always easy either to implement or to stick to. In an ideal world, we would all exclusively breastfeed, not work, stay at home, raise the perfect baby, have a 'proper' family unit, masses of help and support, and never be stressed or overtired. As this is *not* the case for most of us, my plan, although sometimes 'bending the rules' a little, is a down-to-earth and sympathetic approach designed to meet the needs of both parents and baby. It will work for all those who seek a practical and realistic method of babycare.

Mum's the Word . . .

6 Alison's method was always baby-led and mother-focused, working on the basis that if the mother wasn't happy then baby wouldn't be happy either, and vice versa. 9

Y.-L. L.

Sleep, or the lack of it, is probably the most widely written about and discussed topic within the entire range of babycare issues. 'How do I get my baby to sleep through the night?' is the most commonly asked question and sought-after solution among all those who are preparing for or have reached parenthood. It is a pity that such a negative attitude exists towards the whole issue of baby sleep: it suggests that you will have months, possibly years, of interrupted nights, leading to a sleep-deprived, stressful time rather than to an enjoyable, relaxed introduction to life as a family.

By reading this book and following my plan you will learn how to implement a flexible daily feeding and sleeping schedule that will result in your baby being able to sleep 12 hours through the night by around eight weeks old.

> ## Mum's the Word . . .
>
> We followed Alison's sleep plan with our first baby, but if I am completely honest there was a part of me that secretly thought it was a fluke that she slept through the night from six weeks old. However, we now have our third baby and have used Alison's plan for each of our children. Our second slept through at eight weeks and our third at nine weeks. It is definitely *not* a fluke or a coincidence. Our three happy and contented children are living proof that it works!
>
> K. W.

Why is this plan so successful?

There are many child- and babycare books on the market, each offering a different view on the best way of 'bringing up baby'. There was even a television programme of that name, aired on Channel 4 in May 2008, which looked at four different methods of babycare and not only caused a great deal of controversy but, sadly, left many parents even more bewildered about what is the 'right' method to follow. I am loath to bring any more confusion into what seems to be the minefield of parenthood, but I have been persuaded to do so by the hundreds of families who have successfully used my plan. Of course, my plan is based on my own experience, research and opinions, and every parent should take time to consider all the babycare options available before deciding which one is best for them.

With such a lot of advice and help at your fingertips it might seem that parenting today should be an easy experience but, as most methods fail to take into account the individuality of both babies and parents, it can be difficult to adapt and use them within the reality of your own family life. My plan, however, will work for everyone and has already been used successfully by parents with very different circumstances:

- first-time parents
- parents of twins
- single parents
- working mothers
- parents who travel extensively
- teenage mums
- parents of second or subsequent babies
- parents with babies born prematurely
- parents of babies with reflux
- three different sets of triplets
- families from all different cultures
- families of many different religions
- some parents of babies with special needs

Note: Throughout this book I refer at times to 'a partner', 'your husband' or 'daddy' without any intention of alienating single parents or those with other family structures. This plan will work for all, no matter what your individual circumstances.

> ### Mum's the Word . . .
>
> ❛ Alison's plan and her way of establishing a routine were easily tailored to our situation and lifestyle. It wasn't strict or set in stone but sympathetic to our baby and to us as parents. ❜
>
> M. H.

Although the plan is designed to be flexible and encourages you to trust your instincts, it does set out an actual structure and gives step-by-step guidelines. When the word 'routine' is mentioned, many parents automatically think of a strict and prescriptive regime that must be followed to the minute without any deviation. While this is true for the well-known method of babycare set out in *The Contented Little Baby* book, the word 'routine' does not need to be interpreted in this way. If you analyse how most of us live, we do all follow a basic routine of sleep, get up, eat, wash, dress, etc., but with no two days ever being exactly the same and each person's daily routine differing from another's. This is just how it is with babies. They actually respond better if they have a basic routine which follows a particular sequence of daily events, albeit one that may vary slightly from day to day as it incorporates the flexibility of family life.

Many people think that a baby is unable to fall into any sort of routine until around two or three months old. However, I simply don't believe this to be the case. In my experience, the sooner you put a structure in place, the easier it is for both you and your baby to enjoy life as you move through the first few weeks. Babies learn by association almost from the moment they are born, very quickly getting used to whatever is introduced and the conditions surrounding the way they feed and sleep, so whatever you implement in those first few weeks will become the norm for your baby. Trying then to change and introduce something different can often cause confusion and difficulties for both of you. This is why I advise using my plan from Day 1, or at least starting as early as possible.

I have devised the plan to meet all the natural feeding needs and sleeping patterns of any healthy newborn and parents are always amazed at how quickly and easily their baby fits into it – though do remember that all babies are individuals and some fall into the pattern with ease while others can take longer to settle down and need a little more prompting!

By following my plan you will quickly learn whether your baby is crying from hunger, tiredness or some other reason. You will be able to understand and respond to your baby's needs quickly and with confidence, and this will have the knock-on effect of both you and your baby feeling calm, contented and reassured. Within a matter of weeks, as well as having structured daytime naps, your baby will happily go to bed and sleep from around 7pm until 7am without the need for night-time feeds.

So far, I am happy to say that the feedback from people who have followed my plan shows a 100 per cent success rate – and I have even become known by many of them as the 'Magic Sleep Fairy'! Granted, some families have encountered difficulties and setbacks, but all problems have been surmountable owing to the way the plan is formulated, as you will discover through reading this book.

> **Mum's the Word . . .**
>
> ❦ For three days now my baby has slept for 3 hours during the day in one go and is much calmer and happier for it, and it hasn't impacted her night sleep at all. In fact, I think she is sleeping longer during the night now – she is only awake and feeding once at around 2.30am whereas before she was up at 10.30pm and 4.30am. ❦
>
> N. M.

Why have a routine?

As already mentioned, we all follow some sort of routine without even realizing it. Getting out of bed, washing, dressing, eating meals, going to work, taking children to school, shopping, cleaning and so on, right through to going to bed at the end of a day, are all little pockets of routine and within each we follow a similar sequence of actions. The actual events may not be exactly the same from day to day, but we still have our basic 'routine rituals' that keep us on track. If the pattern gets interrupted or disturbed it can throw us out of sync and make us forget for a moment what we should do next! Putting a similar basic daily feeding and sleeping pattern in place for a baby will give him* a sense of security and reassurance.

All babies learn by association. It is therefore important from Day 1 that your baby learns the right associations and how to differentiate between night and day, feeding and cuddling, playing and sleeping. By establishing my plan within the early weeks he will quickly begin to understand and accept the daily sequence of events with regard to his feed and sleep times. This introduces the boundaries which become the mainstay of life and will help to set the precedent for your future parenting. For instance, if from the start you introduce a set sequence of events at the end of each day, this will gradually become an accepted bedtime routine for many years to come.

* Throughout the book I refer to babies as 'he' and 'him'. This is for convenience only and everything of course applies equally to girls.

> ### Alison says . . .
> It is important to remember that any routine should be adaptable and nothing is ever exactly the same from day to day.
> Life is not set in stone and babies are not robots.

It is often thought that young babies know or understand very little of what happens around them. I do not believe this to be true at all: in my opinion a newborn baby is like a sponge, soaking up the influences generated within his environment. Babies learn very quickly and do have minds of their own, often displaying their personality and indicating preferences within the first few weeks of life. It is important for us all to understand exactly how formative the first few years of life actually are. This is beautifully explained in a book called *Why Love Matters* by psychoanalytic psychotherapist Sue Gerdhart.[1] She explains how the human baby is the most socially influenced creature on earth, open from Day 1 to learning what his emotions are and how to manage them. This leads to our earliest experiences as babies having much more relevance to our adult selves than many of us realize. Sue Gerdhart also explores how the earliest relationship can shape a baby's nervous system and how early interactions between babies and their parents will have lasting and serious consequences. She goes on to show how the emotional development of the brain determines future emotional wellbeing and studies the specific early 'pathways' that can affect the way we respond to stress and contribute to conditions such as anorexia, addiction and anti-social behaviour. In my opinion her work and her theories complement and substantiate my ethos and my plan as a sensible and practical approach to looking after your baby.

Implementing this flexible daily sequence of feeding and sleeping will quickly help to build your confidence as a new parent. Be prepared to trust your instincts, believe in your own judgement and enjoy the time you spend with your new baby.

> **Mum's the Word . . .**
>
> ❛ The thing I remember most was being encouraged to think for myself and to trust in my own instincts as a mother, which had been buried under the swamp of conflicting advice that I was bombarded with as a new mum. ❜
>
> M. M.

Questions frequently asked about using a routine

Q   *Why should I follow a routine at all when many other advisers advocate demand feeding?*

A   It is entirely up to each individual to research and then choose their own method of parenting, and undoubtedly each method has its own merits. As you will see from my plan, daytime feeds are very much baby-led, but the decision of when to feed has to come from the parent and not the baby. This leaves parents feeling confident and in control. In my opinion, complete demand feeding is often unmanageable, as parents cannot take charge of their days but are controlled by the demands of the baby. Of course babies have needs which must be met, but if you always assume that need is only for food, then you will never learn to understand the other reasons why your baby may be crying.

> ### *Alison says . . .*
>
> This is a prime example of where my suggestions go against the accepted guidelines, as I do not believe that 'demand feeding' is beneficial to either mother or baby. I fail to understand why parents are encouraged to respond to a 'demand' from a baby in the first few months whereas a 'demand' from a developing toddler is then deemed to be unacceptable behaviour.
>
> Parenting starts from Day 1 and what happens in those

first few months will set the pattern for the future, so surely it is you, the parent, who needs to be the one to put the boundaries in place, rather than your baby?

Q *I want to follow the 'Continuum Concept' for the first four months, then, because I have to return to work when my baby is six months old, I will need to put a routine in place. How can I achieve this?*

A Recently there has been much discussion about this method of babycare. It suggests that you carry your baby in a sling all day, giving him unrestricted access to the breast, and that he sleeps in bed with you at night. A number of parents who use this method do find it works very well for them and fits comfortably into their lifestyle. However, in your case I would strongly advise you to rethink your parenting plan, because to have total contact with your baby for four months and then expect him to accept a complete change of lifestyle will probably be very distressing for both of you. For instance, after sleeping in your bed for four months he will find it difficult to adjust to sleeping in his cot away from your comforting presence. It will be possible to re-train your baby to accept these changes, but in my opinion it would be more realistic to choose a method that you can use from the start without the need for radical change some months later.

Q *We live a very hectic life and travel extensively. How can we manage to put any routine in place?*

A It will be important for your baby to have the security of a feeding and sleeping routine that you can adapt to the changes of your busy life. If you establish my plan within the early weeks, your baby's body clock will be set for sleeping and feeding at regular times, which means that he will easily adapt to other environments. Obviously when travelling across time zones more adjustments will be necessary. For more information on travelling with your baby and how best to cope with time differences, see Chapter 3 (page 92) and Chapter 6 (page 195).

Q   *I work from home and was hoping to put my baby straight on to 4-hourly feeds so that I have more free time during the day. What is your advice on this?*

A   Some babies will readily accept 4-hourly feeds within the first few weeks, but in my experience the hour leading up to feed time is often spent trying to comfort your hungry baby, as a newborn's natural digestive pattern is to feed every 3 hours. Also, putting your baby on a 4-hour feeding pattern too soon could mean that he is unable to take enough milk during the day and therefore may not settle well at bedtime, be hungrier during the night and need night feeds for a longer period of time. If you follow my plan which adopts a 3-hour daytime feeding pattern, it may be slightly more time consuming for the first few weeks, but by around eight weeks your baby could be sleeping 12 hours each night and could be down to 4-hourly feeds by twelve weeks, which in a shorter space of time will give you the freedom you need.

Establishing positive sleep habits and bedtime practice

Over the years, through observation, experience and research, it has become plain to me that young babies are, on the whole, capable of sleeping through the night by around eight weeks of age if the parents follow the simple guidelines detailed in this book. The sooner you start to implement this plan the better, as your baby will not have chance to form any negative sleep associations or bad habits, and will embrace his sleep times now and for many years to come rather than fighting against them.

It is essential for a baby's cognitive and physical development to get enough rest. Without the right amount of sleep your baby may become irritable, fretful, fractious and difficult to feed. During adult sleep, restorative functions occur as the mind and body are given the chance to rest. The same applies to babies, but they also actually grow and develop while they are asleep and it is during this restful period that the majority of actual brain development takes place. In fact, recent research reported in *Nature Neuroscience* indicates that early brain development, learning and memory are all supported by good sleep nutrition, while sleep disruption has been linked to behavioural and emotional problems.[2]

Having worked with hundreds of parents who have implemented my plan, I have personally seen the positive results gained when babies actually get enough sleep within the first few weeks of life. These babies move through their toddler years and into childhood with a healthy, happy and ingrained ability to sleep, and, apart from occasional interruptions to their sleep pattern, continue to be sound sleepers. It is therefore vitally important to ensure that from the beginning your baby develops good sleep habits which you can begin to encourage through a regular bedtime routine and a structured sleep pattern during the day.

> ### *Alison says . . .*
> Most parents are utterly amazed at how much sleep their baby needs and are often misled into thinking that if the baby has less sleep during the day he will sleep better at night. This is simply not the case – actually the opposite will occur, resulting in an overtired baby unable to feed, settle or sleep properly at all.
> Sleep breeds sleep!

The following basic principles should help your baby to develop a healthy association with going to bed and sleep:

○ Learn to understand your baby's sleep patterns and watch for his behavioural signals when he becomes tired.
○ Fostering independent sleep in babies is a positive approach which benefits both the baby and the parents.
○ Put a good bedtime routine in place by following the suggested guidelines as set out in this plan.
○ Ensure your baby has enough good-quality sleep during the day.
○ Spend time with your baby during the day so that he does not seek social interaction during the night.
○ Emphasize the difference between night and day.
○ Provide a good sleep environment in terms of temperature, light, comfort, etc.

○ Where possible, put your baby to bed while he is awake and encourage him to settle himself to sleep for both daytime naps and at night.

○ Avoid responding too quickly to crying while your baby is settling down to sleep. Babies may cry at this time and they often need to be given a chance to settle into sleep by themselves.

○ Ensure your baby is on a good feeding schedule throughout the day and takes sufficient milk.

○ Once you have put your baby down, leave him to wake for his feeds in the night rather than waking him for them.

○ Try not to use any 'sleep aids' – dummy, musical mobiles, constant rocking, patting or rubbing, etc. These could possibly end up being a hindrance to your baby's ability to fall asleep rather than a help, as he may become too dependent on assisted sleep and never learn to fall asleep without his 'aid'.

From the very early days you can start to put some simple procedures in place which your baby will come to recognize as the signals for bedtime. I advise you to introduce them within the first couple of weeks. A possible sequence might be:

 1) Nappy-free time.
 2) Soothing music.
 3) Baby massage.
 4) Bathtime.
 5) A quiet room with lowered lighting.
 6) A bedtime story or song.
 7) Love and cuddles.
 8) The last feed.
 9) A round of 'goodnights'.
10) Bedtime itself.

Whatever steps you decide to introduce, do try to keep to the same sequence and, where possible, include a bath most evenings. Bathtime itself will become the focal point and signal for your baby that bedtime is approaching, and as the years go by this will become the accepted routine: going to bed follows bathtime each night.

Mum's the Word . . .

Before we started to follow Alison's routine we never had any spare time and used to eat our evening meal in shifts so that one of us could see to our baby, who was crying throughout most of the evening. It was only after talking to Alison that we realized our baby was simply overtired and we started putting her to bed each evening at 7pm. It took a few days for her to get used to this, but very soon bedtime couldn't come quickly enough for her and often she would be in bed for 6.30pm and sleep until 7.30am the next day. It was so wonderful to have our evenings back and to be able to sit down to dinner together again. We have even held a dinner party since, and our little girl slept through the whole thing!

S. W.

Sleep cycles

Features of active sleep and quiet sleep	
Active sleep	**Quiet sleep**
Flickering eyelids or even eyes partly open, although your baby is actually still asleep.	Unlikely to be any noticeable eye movement and his eyelids will remain closed.
Arms and legs may twitch or move spasmodically and he may move his head from side to side.	He will be very still with little or no movement of limbs or head.
Breathing may be rapid and irregular and at times he will be taking only small, shallow breaths.	His breathing will become slow, regular and deep.
Facial expressions may change and he may appear to be frowning or smiling.	His whole appearance will be calm and relaxed as he is deeply asleep.

There are two types of sleep: rapid eye movement (REM) sleep and non-rapid eye movement (non-REM) sleep. REM sleep is also known as 'active sleep' and non-REM sleep as 'quiet sleep'. The table on the previous page shows what you might expect to see in your baby during each phase.

The different periods of active and quiet sleep are known as 'sleep cycles' and they are evident in your baby from birth. In adults each sleep cycle runs for approximately 90 minutes, whereas in babies a cycle lasts for around 40 minutes. The first cycle after falling asleep is active sleep, followed by a cycle of quiet sleep, and these continue to alternate through-out the night. As adults we have become used to our sleep patterns and most of us are not aware of the differing cycles through which we pass, but babies who have not yet learned the art of sleep are very sensitive to their sleep cycles. They will often wake after their first 40-minute cycle and can be heard to moan, whimper or even cry for a few minutes before settling themselves back into the next quiet cycle.

These cycles also occur during a baby's daytime naps and it is then even more important to leave him to re-settle himself into quiet sleep without your intervention, thus encouraging structured daytime naps. A baby who does not get enough sleep during the day will become over-tired and irritable and this will then hinder his ability to settle down to sleep for the night.

> ### *Alison says . . .*
>
> It is often lack of understanding of these sleep cycles that can lead parents and their babies into the problems of continually disturbed nights, no regular daytime naps and therefore ongoing sleep deprivation.

Because a baby learns by association, if he is given immediate atten-tion when he stirs throughout his sleep he will not be able to develop the ability to re-settle himself after waking during his natural sleep cycles.

One of the more common problems which parents ask me to solve is that their baby will sleep for only 40 minutes at a time, especially during the day. To encourage him to develop a positive sleep pattern, if your baby does wake and cry out after he has been asleep for 40 minutes or so, try to be patient and leave him for a few minutes to see if he will settle himself back to sleep. I do appreciate that this is one of the hardest things to do for any new parent, as your natural instinct is to comfort your baby as soon as he stirs, but if you can manage to follow this advice the rewards will soon be evident and your baby will be able to sleep for as long as he needs.

This rule applies to both daytime naps and nighttime sleeping and it can be hard to follow in either case, but for different reasons:

Daytime naps

- It can be difficult to believe that after your baby has had 40 minutes or so of sleep he can still be tired and need to sleep for longer.
- As a new parent you want to cuddle your baby as much as possible and find it hard even to put him down for a nap, let alone leave him if he cries a little.
- Friends and relatives will be visiting in the early weeks and want to have cuddles with your new baby, regardless of whether it is nap time or not, so as soon as he stirs you may be encouraged to pick him up even though he may actually still need more sleep.
- After your baby has been asleep for a short time it may be tempting to pick him up as soon as he stirs because you need to go out, but it would be better to put your baby in his pram, ready to go out, for the whole of nap time, rather than letting him sleep for just a short while and then disturbing him.

Nighttime sleep

- Any whimper or moan, let alone a cry, is amplified at night when everything else is so quiet and so it sounds so much worse.
- You may be worried that the baby will wake other children if he is not picked up straight away.
- Many of the sound monitors on the market today flash red lights at the first few sounds a baby makes. This looks very alarming and may encourage you to react hastily and unnecessarily.

○   When a baby is sleeping in his parent's room Mum may tend to him as soon as he makes a noise to prevent waking Dad, who has to get up for work in the morning.

Mum's the Word . . .

❝ I found it so hard to leave my baby crying even for a few seconds and I felt like I was the worst mother in the world. Even though I never left her for more than a few minutes or so each time, it was still really difficult. But I am so pleased that I followed Alison's advice. My baby learned how to sleep through the night in the first few weeks and is now a complete 'sleep monster' – she actually looks forward to taking her naps and loves going to bed at night. ❞

J. H.

Questions frequently asked about sleep

Q   *I have been given a lovely mobile to go over the cot. What is your advice on using these?*

A   I have always been amazed at the number of toys and cot mobiles on the market today that are advertised as 'sleep aids' for babies. In fact I have found nearly all of them to be more stimulating than soothing, which means they may have the adverse effect of keeping your baby awake rather than helping him drift off to sleep. Another possible problem is that if your baby gets so used to hearing and watching a mobile as he does go to sleep, he will very soon rely on it as a 'crutch' for sleep and throughout his natural night-waking in the early weeks he may need it turned on again and again. See Chapter 3 for further information on sleep associations.

Q   *Surely my baby will just fall asleep when he is tired, so why do I need to follow any set sleep routine?*

A   It does seem to be a crazy phenomenon that babies will not just fall asleep when they are tired, but in my experience they simply do not! Sleep does not seem to come naturally to them and, having been 'nocturnal' in the womb, after birth they actually have to learn the art of sleeping. Babies who become overtired find it even harder to fall asleep and this can easily become a vicious circle of baby being overtired but still unable to sleep well. In order to encourage their sleep patterns to develop, I believe it is necessary to provide suitable surroundings, regular feeds and a simple bed-time routine. Babies do need a lot of sleep in the early months, and they need to sleep during the day as well as at night, so my advice is to have some structure to each day which will lead to regular nap times. You can achieve this by following the plan set out in this book.

Q *I have a very noisy house with two older children, a dog and a husband who is an avid and vocal football supporter. How can I expect my new baby to sleep through any of this?*
A   Many parents worry that ordinary daytime noise will wake their baby during nap times, but actually this is rarely the case. Your baby will already have become accustomed to the noises within your home while he was in the womb, therefore after he is born he should not be too disturbed by them when he is sleeping. Obviously it is advisable to tone down excessive noise where possible and it helps if you put the baby in his room and close the door for nap times. Many parents go to unnecessary lengths to reduce or eliminate the sounds that are normally heard in their environment while their baby is sleeping, but it is not essential to do so and there need not be any restrictions on your daily way of life.

Sleep deprivation in babies

Very few people realize that babies can actually suffer from sleep deprivation. It is estimated that half of all infants in Western societies are getting less sleep than they should – usually falling short by at least 2 hours in every 24 (see Chapter 3). According to the Sleep in America Poll, carried out annually by the National Sleep Foundation task force, the rate of sleep deprivation has increased in recent years and is a trend that continues to climb.[3]

This comes as no surprise to me: I have encountered first-hand the increasing numbers of parents who are seeking help to get their babies sleeping through the night. They often contact me at the point of sheer exhaustion and complete desperation after months of little or no sleep because their babies continually wake throughout the night. I believe that sleep problems in babies are escalating due to a number of factors:

- The advice that babies should sleep in the parents' bedroom for at least the first six months.
- Since the introduction of the Back-to-Sleep Campaign the advice regarding sleep position has been changed and most babies are now placed on their backs to sleep. However, many babies struggle to relax and settle into sleep in this unnatural position.
- Babies who suffer from gastro-oesophageal reflux will generally be more uncomfortable when laid flat on their backs and will often be unable to sleep (see Chapter 7).
- Many parents follow babycare methods that require them to wake their baby during the late evening to give what has become known as the 'dream feed', thus disturbing their baby's developing natural sleep pattern (see Chapters 3 and 6).
- It is becoming increasingly understood and accepted that many women are now having babies later in life. These older mums often experience higher levels of anxiety and are less likely to be able to leave their babies to settle to sleep without feeling the need to check on them constantly. This may ultimately instigate feelings of anxiety in their newborns and disturb their developing sleep habits.

It has long since been proved that sleep deprivation in babies takes a toll on their development and, if not resolved, sleep disturbances that start in infancy can continue into late childhood. A long-term study in the *Journal of Child Psychology and Psychiatry* shows how infants who suffered from chronic sleep deprivation were much more likely at five and ten years old to be still suffering from sleep problems than were children who slept well as babies. This lack of sleep has a knock-on negative effect on their physical and emotional health and also on their behaviour as they grow up. See Chapters 3 and 6 for further information on sleep deprivation and its effects.

> **Mum's the Word . . .**
>
> ❧ We were shocked when we discovered that our baby was
> simply overtired and the previous behaviours that we thought
> were 'cute' – having 'itchy' feet, or being able to say 'no' by
> thrashing his head at the age of four months – were in fact
> signs of stress due to him being completely sleep-deprived.
> We thought we had one of those babies that just doesn't need
> much sleep, but after following Alison's advice our baby
> turned into the best sleeper ever. At ten months he was still
> sleeping around 16 hours out of every 24 and is now such a
> happy, calm and contented little boy. ❧
>
> I. T.

Sleep deprivation in parents

It is estimated that as adults we spend one third of our lives in bed, though
the amount of sleep an adult needs does vary from person to person and
also from one developmental state to another. According to researchers, an
adult needs on average around 7.5–8 hours of unbroken, good-quality
sleep each night. When a new baby arrives, the parents' sleep is inevitably
disrupted and it is estimated that they can easily lose about 200 hours of
sleep during their child's first year.

Long-term sleep deprivation can have far-reaching effects on our
physical, mental and emotional wellbeing. Symptoms include:

- an increase in digestive disorders
- an increase in cardiovascular problems
- slower reactions and physical reflexes
- difficulty with sight and problems focusing
- heightened sensitivity to pain
- tendency to mood swings
- increased irritability and lack of patience
- inability to stay alert and vigilant

○ difficulty in controlling emotions
○ loss of concentration and inability to 'think straight'
○ headaches and migraines
○ impaired memory and lack of logical thinking
○ increased risk of suffering from depression and anxiety disorders

Looking at that list, it is a wonder that anyone who suffers from any of the symptoms of sleep deprivation can ever manage to look after themselves – let alone a new baby!

I would like to emphasize here the importance of the last point: the increased risk of experiencing some form of depression. Sleep deprivation is actually a major factor in post-natal depression (PND). Thankfully, many mums with whom I have worked who were either displaying symptoms of or had been diagnosed with PND gradually began to see an improvement in their symptoms as the sleep issues with their babies were resolved and everyone was able to get some much-needed rest. See also Chapters 3, 6 and 7 for more on sleep deprivation, sleep-training and reflux.

Did You Know?

Post-natal depression (PND) is a recognized and treatable illness which affects approximately 15–20 per cent of mothers and 10 per cent of fathers. (In fathers it is not classed as actual PND, but these men do suffer from a similar type of depression.)

It may come on immediately after the arrival of the baby but can also present itself later, or go unrecognized (especially by the mother herself) for weeks or months.

Many mothers often feel anxious, tearful and unable to look forward to anything, sometimes can be irritable, feel very despondent and suffer extreme fatigue.

They may have a sense of inadequacy and feelings of failure, and often experience physical symptoms such as headaches and lethargy.

It is common for a mother to believe that she is unable to cope and to have irrational fears, possibly feeling that things won't ever be the same as they were before. It is important to remember that it is the depression that makes her feel like this and that she will recover from PND, although it may take time.

For more information and advice on PND, contact Liz Wise, a specialist post-natal depression counsellor and trainer with a diploma in humanistic counselling:
www.postnataldepression.com

☆ *Alison's Golden Rules* ☆

1 Keep following my Sensational Baby Sleep Plan to ensure that neither you nor your baby will experience any long-term sleep deprivation.

2 Do be aware that babies actually respond better to being in a routine – albeit a flexible one – of feed and sleep times.

3 Do remember that sleep breeds sleep, and the more sleep your baby gets, the better.

4 Remember that babies can easily get overtired and often need more sleep than you think.

5 Babies are not born with negative sleep associations, they only learn and adopt the bad habits we teach them.

6 Understand that babies who learn to sleep well during the early months are less likely to experience long-term sleep problems.

7 Ensure that you are providing the appropriate surroundings and atmosphere to promote healthy sleep associations from the start.

8 Do remember that daytime naps can take slightly longer to get established than the long sleep throughout the night.

9 Have faith that your baby is capable of sleeping 12 hours through the night by around eight weeks of age.

10 Enjoy these first few weeks with your baby: they are very special and will all too soon be just a memory – hopefully a happy one and not a nightmare!

2

Feeding

How you should feed your baby is a much-discussed topic that arouses strong feelings, firm opinions and often judgemental views from all those involved – and even from those who are not! Everyone has an opinion and will eagerly share it with you, even though you may not wish to hear what they have to say or to follow the advice they offer.

In an ideal world, all mothers would be able to give birth naturally, the baby would latch on to the breast straight away and continue to breastfeed successfully without any problems at all. Sadly, this is not the case for the majority of mothers. We all know, and are certainly told often enough, that 'breast is best', but in my view it is better to adopt an approach that can be adapted to your lifestyle than to restrict yourself to a method that you may find difficult to maintain.

Alison says . . .

I promote and support breastfeeding, but never to the detriment of mother or baby.

In my opinion there should be no pressure on any mother to make the supposed 'right' choice, as stated in the currently accepted guidelines, nor

Mum's the Word . . .

My baby was not gaining weight, I was really struggling with breastfeeding and my baby never slept. Alison came round and after much discussion we gave Margot her first bottle of formula. She sucked it down in 1 minute flat and then fell asleep for 3 hours. It was a beautiful sunny day – the first time I had noticed in three weeks. I had a feeling of complete relief and physically felt my shoulders loosen as the tension flooded out of me. I realized that formula feeding was not 'evil' and bad, and that, as Alison had said, 'a happy mum makes a happy baby'. Margot and I have never looked back . . . Breast is best, but not for everyone!

C. B-W.

any stigma attached to her ability or to her decision to breastfeed or not. It is up to each individual to research the facts, take into consideration the guidelines in place, then trust her own judgement about the method of feeding that is right for her baby, her family, her lifestyle and herself.

Which method of feeding?

The guidelines from the World Health Organization advise that exclusive breastfeeding for the first six months is now recommended. However, for many mothers this may not actually be achievable, either through choice, circumstance or inability. In my opinion it is better to take a more realistic view, to weigh up the pros and cons and to find the way forward that suits each individual mother and baby. This decision may be influenced by many different factors, including:

- Your own emotions and feelings. Some mothers have a set plan to breastfeed exclusively, while others just hate the whole idea.
- Lack of practical support and advice, giving rise to feelings of uncertainty about what to do for the best.
- Pressure from a partner who either insists that you should breastfeed because he believes it to be best, or insists that you bottlefeed so that he can help feed the baby.
- Having to return to work during the first year and needing the flexibility of introducing bottlefeeding.
- It may not be your first baby and with other lively children to deal with you may have less time to concentrate on breastfeeding.
- Jealousy from a demanding toddler who is upset with a new baby.
- Other family matters, such as a bereavement, that take your time and focus away from being able to breastfeed.
- Previous breast surgery that may now affect your ability to breastfeed and/or to produce milk.
- Possible reluctance to breastfeed if you feel uncomfortable at the prospect of feeding in public or in company.
- A busy or hectic lifestyle that may mean having to leave your baby with other people from time to time.

○   The cost of the extra equipment and formula needed for bottlefeeding, with the added inconvenience of having to wash and sterilize the equipment.

There are many factors in your life that may affect your decision about which method of feeding to adopt. The following lists show some advantages for each method.

Exclusive breastfeeding

○   Breast milk is designed to be more easily digested by the baby's sensitive and still developing digestive system.
○   Breast milk contains less sodium and protein than formula.
○   There is less risk of a breastfed baby developing allergies such as asthma or eczema later in life.
○   As breast milk is a natural food source, it is unlikely that a breastfed baby will suffer from constipation or diarrhoea.
○   Breast milk is high in antibodies, which during the first few weeks will enhance the baby's immune system.
○   Breast milk is nearly always readily available and served at the right temperature.
○   Breastfeeding assists the recovery of the mother by helping the uterus to contract to its normal size.

Breastfeeding and expressing breast milk

All the above reasons, plus:

○   Introducing your baby to a bottle early enough can prevent a later rejection.
○   Other people can sometimes help with a feed.
○   You can express some milk before going to bed and have a longer rest while Daddy gives a night feed.
○   Expressing can help to stimulate your milk supply.
○   If your baby is ill or in special care and unable to breastfeed, he can still have your expressed breast milk.

○ Some babies with reflux can still have expressed breast milk when fed through a bottle with added feed thickeners and medication.
○ If you are ill or have to go into hospital and can't breastfeed for any length of time, your baby will be used to taking a bottle.
○ If you need to take medication that isn't healthy for your baby, you can express your milk and throw it away to ensure a healthy future supply.
○ If your nipples are sore you can express the milk to maintain supply while 'resting' them.
○ You may have twins or triplets and need to express so that each baby can be fed with some breast milk.
○ If you are not breastfeeding throughout the night you can have an alcoholic drink or two in the evening, then express and discard your milk before you go to bed.

Breastfeeding combined with formula feeding

All the reasons from both the above lists, plus:

○ A hungry baby may need extra sustenance from some formula to help maintain a healthy weight gain.
○ If you are anxious about breastfeeding in public you have the flexibility of doing that at home and formula feeding when out.
○ A baby of large birth weight may benefit from being 'topped-up' with formula if breast milk alone is not sufficient to satisfy his hunger.
○ If you do not like to – or even cannot – express your milk but still want to have the flexibility of mixed feeding, then you can give formula as well as breast milk.
○ By introducing a formula feed in the early weeks, if for any reason your milk supply decreases or you suddenly cannot breastfeed, you should have no problem changing to formula feeding.

Exclusive formula feeding

There are some very real advantages to formula feeding and sometimes it is really necessary to do so:

○ It is easier to monitor milk intake and see how much your baby drinks.

○ Formula gives longer and more lasting satisfaction to a baby.

○ Babies with a lactose intolerance can be fed a lactose-free formula.

○ Babies with either a cow's-milk protein intolerance and/or multiple food allergies can be fed with hypoallergenic formulas designed specifically for babies with these problems.

○ Some babies who suffer with reflux respond better to specially designed anti-reflux formulas than to breast milk.

○ Siblings can be more involved and 'help' at feed times, hopefully initiating more interaction and acceptance of the new baby.

○ More freedom for the mother, avoiding the feeling that you are only used as a 'feeding machine'.

○ Your partner can have much more involvement with feeding your baby from the start.

○ Less physical and emotional strain than on a mother who is breastfeeding.

○ More freedom with your choice of clothes as you do not need easy access to your breasts at all times!

○ Fewer dietary restrictions and demands on the mother.

○ It is safe for you to take antibiotics or other medication as these will not transfer into your baby through your milk.

○ No interference from sore or leaking breasts when resuming sexual relations.

Understanding breastfeeding

Breastfeeding is a skill that doesn't necessarily come naturally and needs to be learned by both mother and baby. All women are different, breasts and nipples come in all shapes and sizes, and babies are complete individuals. Therefore every woman's breastfeeding experience will be different from the next and while some will cope with ease, others will never feel comfortable with breastfeeding and won't particularly enjoy it.

There is a very good book by Clare Byam-Cook called *What to Expect*

When Breastfeeding . . . And What If You Can't?, which is, in my view, the best and most comprehensive guide to the subject.[4] It explains how to breast-feed and gives practical advice to help overcome all the issues that go along with it in far greater detail than I have space to do in this book. However, the following sections should give you a basic knowledge and provide enough information to help you breastfeed successfully.

First, here are brief explanations of some terms commonly used in connection with breastfeeding.

Progesterone   A hormone that causes a change to occur in the uterus in the latter part of each menstrual cycle and is also present in higher levels throughout pregnancy.

Oestrogen   Another hormone, but one that promotes and maintains female body characteristics. Both progesterone and oestrogen are known as the 'maternal hormones' and it is their presence in a newborn baby of either sex that can cause the mammary tissue to swell temporarily, occasionally even producing a white fluid known as 'witch's milk'. These breast swellings will disappear without treatment as the hormone levels in the baby decrease.

Oxytocin   A pituitary hormone that is released into the body and is responsible for the muscle contractions during labour. It also works on the breast muscles during lactation to instigate the release of milk from the internal ducts. Synthetic preparations of this hormone are called Pitocin or Syntocinon and are used to induce or accelerate labour.

Alison says . . .

It is rarely mentioned that when breastfeeding you may experience a feeling similar to sexual arousal. This is entirely normal, so don't worry! It is simply caused by the hormone oxytocin contracting your uterine muscles, which is a similar process to the one that instigates an orgasm.

Prolactin A hormone that is produced at the same time as oxytocin but which actually triggers the production of milk and continues to stimulate the milk glands to maintain a regular flow.

Lactation This term is applied to both the production and the secretion of milk during the breastfeeding process.

Let-down reflex This is caused by the release of prolactin, which then stimulates the breasts to produce more milk. While a baby is suckling this is an ongoing process and some mothers actually feel a warm, tingling sensation in their breasts when the hormone takes effect and the breasts empty and re-fill.

Nipples These vary in size, colour and position, but all contain two types of muscle fibres. These are circular, sphincter-like muscle fibres which surround the ducts, and erective, erogenous muscle fibres which lie alongside the ducts. These muscles respond to cold, touch and stimulation. Most commonly nipples stand out from the areola (see below), but around 10 per cent of women have flat or inverted nipples. See pages 54–9 on problems with breastfeeding.

Areola The pink or brown circular area that surrounds the nipple, behind which are the glandular lobes that will become the milk reservoirs during the lactation period. On the surface of the areola are the special sebaceous glands known as Montgomery's Tubercles. These are thought to secrete an antibacterial sebum which keeps the nipples moist and provides a protective film during pregnancy and lactation.

Colostrum During the latter stage of pregnancy and directly after birth the body produces the first milk, known as colostrum. It is often bright yellow and thick, and usually only a small amount is produced, although this should be enough to sustain the baby until the milk comes in. Colostrum contains a high level of protein to nourish a new baby and also acts as a laxative which helps his digestive system to pass the thick meconium that is present in the intestine while a baby is in the womb. Over two or three days the colostrum is gradually replaced by the production of breast milk.

Foremilk   When a baby starts to feed at the breast it is mainly foremilk that is produced. This is high in volume, helps to quench the baby's thirst and increases his fluid intake. Foremilk is also high in lactose (a milk-sugar), proteins and other essential vitamins and antibodies to promote growth and help to resist infection. Foremilk is often very watery in appearance and can be a pale-blue, blue or grey colour.

Hind-milk   After the baby has been at the breast for some minutes, feeding slows and this leads to the production of hind-milk. This is less in quantity than the foremilk and has a much higher fat and calorific content which helps to sustain and satisfy the baby for longer. Hind-milk has a quite thick consistency and is usually a rich, creamy yellow or white colour.

> ### Alison says . . .
> If you express your breast milk and leave it to stand in the fridge for a few hours you will notice the difference between the foremilk and the hind-milk. The fat-rich hind-milk will settle and form a creamy layer on top of the foremilk, as can be seen in an ordinary bottle of full-fat cow's milk.

How breasts work

If you are planning to breastfeed it may help you to understand the actual anatomy of breasts and the physiological changes that occur in them during the last stage of pregnancy, through labour and after the birth.

The breasts during pregnancy
○   They may become enlarged as they are stimulated by progesterone, causing the milk ducts to increase in size.
○   There may be a tingling sensation and a feeling of fullness and heaviness.
○   They may secrete a few drops of colostrum throughout pregnancy but, due to the high levels of oestrogen and progesterone, actual milk production will not usually occur until after the birth.

○   The areola may become darker in appearance, possibly to help the baby focus on it as he searches for the nipple.
○   The nipple may become slightly larger.

The breasts during and after labour

○   As labour progresses, the levels of oestrogen and progesterone drop significantly to allow the production of oxytocin and prolactin which are essential to stimulate both birth and the start of milk production.
○   Following the delivery of the placenta the increasing levels of prolactin begin to act on the breasts to stimulate milk production, even though the baby may not be suckling.
○   Prolactin will continue to stimulate milk production for around ten days, then will gradually decrease if the mother is not breastfeeding or expressing.

The breasts after giving birth

○   Initially the breasts will produce colostrum as a first food until true milk production begins at around Day 3.
○   As the breasts fill up and are then emptied by the baby's suckling, the composition of the breast milk changes from foremilk to hind-milk throughout each feed.
○   Gradually the level of hormones will even out and the milk supply is then mainly stimulated by the baby suckling at the breast.
○   It can take between six and eight weeks for breastfeeding to become established, during which time the breasts become accustomed to producing the amount of milk the baby needs for each feed.
○   During the first few weeks the milk supply is regulated by the amount taken or expressed at each feed rather than by the release of prolactin alone.
○   While breastfeeding, some mothers may actually feel the let-down reflex as a warm, tingling – sometimes even painful – sensation in the breasts.
○   Due to the increased level of oxytocin during breast stimulation, some mothers may feel stomach cramps or 'mini contractions' which are due to the action of the hormone on the uterus, helping it to contract to its original size.

The emotional aspect

The extent of hormonal changes occurring in your body during lactation means it can be an extremely emotional time. When you put your baby to the breast a message is sent via the nervous system to the hypothalamus in the brain which then stimulates the production of oxytocin and prolactin to encourage milk production. However, the hypothalamus, being the 'seat of emotions', can react adversely and suppress the production of these hormones if you are feeling stressed, overtired, anxious or tense. Understanding this emotional cycle may help you to continue breastfeeding successfully by knowing when to take a break, whether perhaps to supplement a feed with either expressed milk or formula, and when to get some much-needed rest.

Questions frequently asked about breastfeeding

Q   *How often should I put my baby to the breast in the first few days?*
A   In the first few days after birth your breasts will produce colostrum and, because of the small amounts produced and the fact that a new-born baby can be very sleepy, new mothers often do not realize the importance of frequently putting the baby to the breast. I advise that instead of letting your baby 'demand' when to feed, in these early days you should wake him and put him to the breast every 2–3 hours during the day, then leave him to sleep and feed him only when he wakes during the night. Do offer both breasts: though he may suckle for only 5–10 minutes on each side, first, this should ensure that he gets sufficient nourishment and hydration; second, it will encourage and stimulate your milk production; and third, the colostrum will aid the expulsion of the meconium from your baby's digestive system.

Q   *I am having a planned Caesarean section. Will this affect my ability to breastfeed?*
A   No, it should not, and because most operations are carried out using a spinal tap rather than a general anaesthetic you should be able to put your baby to your breast reasonably quickly after birth. One slight

drawback can be that your milk may take a little longer to come in, as during a planned, artificial birth the hormones are not active in the birth process. However, for anyone needing an emergency C-section after the onset of labour this will not be the case, as the hormones will have initiated the birth process and so will already be present.

Q   *I have had breast-reduction surgery and my nipples had to be re-sited. Will I be able to breastfeed?*
A   In truth, there is no way of telling whether you will be able to breast-feed or not until you try. In many cases the nipples, muscle receptors, nerves and milk ducts are undamaged by the procedure and therefore breastfeeding is possible, but, sadly, for others this may not be the case. If your nipples have returned to a near normal level of sensation all may be well, but if you have lost sensation since the operation then it is likely that there has been a degree of nerve damage affecting the necessary stimulation for the onset of lactation. Breast reduction or enlargement alone, without interference to the nipple, rarely decreases the ability of a mother to breastfeed.

Breastfeeding basics

Milk supply and production

Most breastfeeding mothers worry about whether they are producing an adequate supply of milk. This is a real concern for women which should not be dismissed as a trivial matter by health professionals and other advisers.

The amount of colostrum taken by a baby in the first 24 hours is approximately 7.5ml per feed. This gradually increases during the next few days to around 70ml on Day 5. The volume and rate of increase may depend on the frequency of feeding and the ability of your baby to feed well, some becoming more efficient at breastfeeding than others.

During the first few days after birth it may be difficult for you as a new mother to believe that your breasts will produce sufficient nourish-ment for your baby. They may still be soft and unchanged, and you may not see any evidence of colostrum production. Today's guidelines do not advocate giving any milk supplements to your baby during this early stage, but I suggest that each new mother and baby should be treated as the individuals that they are and each situation assessed accordingly. If you feel that your baby is hungry, unsettled and crying even after having what you assume to be a substantial feed at the breast, don't be afraid to offer a supplementary feed if you feel you need to do so.

The amount of milk that is produced varies greatly between individual mothers, but most will normally make more milk than their baby actually takes. There is no doubt that 'supply and demand' is a fundamental factor in sustaining milk supply and your baby does need to be put to the breast at regular intervals to maintain this. Each time your breast is drained, your milk supply is replenished and increased. If you follow the three-hour plan as explained in Chapter 4, this should ensure a successful breastfeeding schedule and maintain your milk supply.

A healthy newborn baby should be able to feed well at the breast and then last for a couple of hours between feeds. If your baby seems unable to do this, then there are many things that you will need to check – see pages 54–9 for advice on feeding difficulties.

Alison says . . .

Do remember that if you are struggling with your breastfeeding, feeling under pressure and are beginning to dread each feed, there is always another option. You have the right to choose and try out another method without being made to feel guilty.

Milk insufficiency

Milk insufficiency is the most common reason for mothers to decide to give up breastfeeding. This fact reflects not only the general lack of confidence that mothers have in their ability to provide sufficient milk for their babies, but also – and more importantly – a lack of support and practical advice which, if available, might help many to overcome the difficulty. Other common problems with which many breastfeeding mothers struggle are: an inability to achieve a good position or latch; becoming so overtired that the quantity and/or quality of their breast milk are affected; being given poor advice on a feeding schedule; the suggestion to feed on demand; or a digestive problem, such as reflux, from which the baby may be suffering. Once these problems have been eliminated, most breastfeeding mothers should be able to produce a sufficient supply. There are, however, others who are physiologically unable to breastfeed or genuinely unable to produce sufficient milk for their babies, and these mothers will be able to substitute formula for breast milk to feed and nurture their babies.

Engorgement

During the first week after giving birth, your milk production will begin whether you are going to breastfeed or not. Some women find this happens relatively quickly and, almost overnight, their breasts become enlarged, feel hot and can be quite painful. For others the milk comes in at a more gradual rate and they escape the discomfort of engorgement. If your breasts do become very full and quite hard, this may cause the nipples to flatten and make it difficult for your baby to latch on, so it may be necessary for you to alleviate the problem by expressing a little milk before offering the breast. You can express either by using a pump or by hand. It is rare for engorgement of the breasts to occur at other times as long as your baby is feeding well, emptying your breasts on a regular basis, and you are following a structured feeding plan.

Care of yourself while breastfeeding

So much in 'mother-care' has changed during the last century that today's new mothers have a very different experience of childbirth and breastfeeding from that of their great-great-grandmothers:

○   Over a hundred years ago a mother would have had her baby
    delivered at home by the local midwife, who would then move into
    the household for around two to four weeks to help the mother,

who was expected to stay in bed during this time, known as her 'lying-in' period.

○ Sixty to seventy years ago a mother could easily have spent around two weeks in hospital after giving birth, with further support at home from a community midwife, and during that time would have had hands-on help to get breastfeeding established.

○ Thirty to forty years ago a mother typically spent seven days in hospital after giving birth and then had daily visits from the midwife for a further two weeks or so, during which time any problems with breastfeeding could be identified and corrected.

○ Today a mother spends as little as 12–48 hours in hospital after giving birth and is lucky to have two or three visits from a midwife before being discharged from their care at around Day 10!

Add to this the fact that most new parents today unfortunately do not have the help and support of members of the extended family, who would once have been close at hand but are now often spread around the globe, and you have a situation in which a new mother is left to struggle on her own with little or no support. It is no wonder that so many find the pressure to exclusively breastfeed their babies on demand for the first six months almost impossible to manage.

To help you through the first few weeks, my advice is to enlist as much practical help as possible from anyone who offers it. If friends and neighbours ask if there is anything they can do for you, don't be too hasty to dismiss their offers with polite thanks but take them up on it – don't be shy! It may be they can cook a meal or two, do some shopping, help with the housework or ironing, or even look after your baby for an hour or two so you can have a break. Granted, childbirth is supposed to be a natural phase in your life, but today there are so many pressures on women to be the perfect wife and mother, to be a complete 'domestic goddess' alongside managing a brilliant career. Remember: you don't have to be superwoman and it is OK to accept as much help as you can get – it doesn't mean you are a failure in any way.

Mum's the Word . . .

I had been given Alison's number by a friend, but I was determined I was going to cope. We had been trying for a baby for so long and now she was finally here, I was sure it would all be a 'natural breeze'. However, six weeks in we were almost wishing we hadn't even had her . . . it was a complete nightmare. Breastfeeding was horrendous, I was absolutely exhausted, the baby never slept, my husband was also so stressed and tired, and we were rowing all the time. I finally picked up the phone and called Alison, but I felt like a complete failure at having to ask for help. What was wrong with me? Why couldn't I manage like every other mother? I felt that I was utterly useless as a mother and would never be able to get it right.

During her visit Alison implemented a brilliant feeding and sleeping schedule that worked for us and our baby. I carried on mainly breastfeeding but introduced two bottlefeeds of either expressed milk or formula each day. Our baby began to sleep properly – it was wonderful. Also, after Alison's 'marriage-guidance-counsellor role' while she stayed with us, we were able to understand each other's feelings and express our own, which stopped the rows and helped our relationship get back on track too. We have never looked back and will always fondly remember the time Alison spent with us.   S. W.

Diet and fluid intake

An important part of successful breastfeeding is making sure that you have a healthy balanced diet with plenty of fluids. While breastfeeding you will need on average an extra 500 calories a day and it is vital that you drink as much water as possible. Some mothers find they have a natural thirst which prompts them to drink more, while others easily forget, so my advice is to make sure that you always have a large glass or bottle of water to hand each time you settle down to a feed. A breastfeeding mum can easily become dehydrated through lack of fluids and often the first sign of this can be a pounding headache.

Eating healthy (and sometimes unhealthy!) snacks between meals is also a good way of keeping up your blood-sugar levels and increasing your intake of calories. What you should eat remains a completely individual choice and I usually advise continuing with the same balanced diet that you ate throughout your pregnancy. It is an extremely good idea to stock up your freezer with home-cooked meals a few weeks in advance to save time once your new baby has arrived; you can also stock up on healthy and easy-to-eat snacks. All the different food groups are important while breastfeeding, so a varied diet that includes fresh fruit and vegetables, some protein and carbohydrate is advisable. I have, however, known many mums who are so busy looking after the baby that they struggle even to grab a banana during the day, let alone eat three balanced meals and healthy snacks, but generally they still manage to produce breast milk. So don't get too anxious and put yourself under even more pressure if you find that biscuits, sweets, ready meals or even take-aways are the only things you have time to eat for a while.

It can be advisable to continue to take your pre-natal mineral and vitamin supplements, as they also help to boost your general health while you are breastfeeding.

Certain foods can have a negative effect on some babies and may cause them to be unsettled, have bouts of crying, become very 'windy' and have explosive stools, or even vomit. If possible, try to monitor your diet in relation to your baby's behaviour to see if you can pinpoint whether a particular food is causing this type of reaction. You can then eliminate it from your diet while breastfeeding. In general, foods that seem to cause problems in some babies are:

- strawberries and raspberries
- onions, peppers, chillies and hot spices
- spicy and very rich, cream-based curries
- citrus fruit and juices
- caffeine, which is found in tea, chocolate and fizzy drinks, not just coffee

○   alcohol (especially champagne, as the bubbles almost seem to transfer into the breast milk – result: one very bloated and windy baby!)

Most foods, even those listed above, are OK in moderation, but it is easy to 'overdose' on one food without realizing it. For instance, a bowl of tomato soup followed by a salad containing fresh tomatoes at lunchtime, then pasta with a bolognese sauce for supper and you have consumed a large quantity of tomatoes in one day which is more than likely to cause some digestive discomfort within your baby.

If you have an alcoholic drink the alcohol content will peak within your breast milk between 60 and 90 minutes afterwards. Once your baby is sleeping through, or you are supplementing night feeds with expressed milk or formula, you can safely have a drink or two in the evening and feed your baby the next morning without any cause for concern. However, if you do happen to have more than one or two drinks, then it is advisable to express your breast milk before you go to bed and discard it, as it will contain a high level of toxins from the alcohol.

Some babies are sensitive or even allergic to cow's-milk protein and/or lactose which is in their mother's breast milk. These problems are explained in detail in Chapter 7.

Positioning and the 'latch'

Correct positioning and getting a good 'latch' are often the keys to successful breastfeeding. Your midwife should offer some hands-on help. Before you are discharged from the community team do make sure you are confident and feel comfortable that breastfeeding is becoming established and that your baby is feeding well. You may be referred to or ask to see a breastfeeding counsellor if things are not going well and they may well be of help, but I would still advise you to read the section further on in this chapter, 'breastfeeding problems', pages 54–9, and Chapter 7, which may help explain why you are experiencing real difficulties.

It will undoubtedly take time for you to find the position which is most comfortable for you and your baby, and a certain amount of trial and error will occur during the first week or so. Try different chairs, the sofa, sitting up on a bed and using pillows or cushions to find where you are most comfortable. Many parents buy a 'rocking-feeding' chair and footstool, but in my experience these are totally unnecessary, extremely expensive and not very practical. When you are feeding your baby, the last thing you need is for him to be rocked to sleep, which will often happen as you rock to and fro in these chairs. In the early weeks it can be hard enough to keep your baby awake and alert enough throughout a feed without the rocking motion which induces sleep. Also, these chairs can quickly become redundant as many mums discover that there is not enough room on either side to fit their ever-growing baby comfortably into a good breastfeeding position.

The following points take you step by step through a breastfeed and should help you find a suitable and comfortable position, which will in turn help you achieve a good latch.

- Wherever you sit, ensure that you have good support for your back.
- Try to make sure you are feeling as calm and relaxed as possible – though with sore nipples, the thought of anyone coming near your boobs, let alone getting baby latched on, can make it impossible to feel relaxed!
- Have an assortment of pillows or cushions close by in case you need them.
- Keep a glass or bottle of water within reach.
- Have some snacks to hand in case you get hungry – most breastfed babies get used to being covered in crumbs!
- Make sure the phone or TV remote are within reach in case you need them.
- Try to sit back and relax your shoulders. I see so many mums who are tense and hunch forward, which puts strain on the back and neck.
- If sitting in a chair, ideally your legs should be high enough to make a 90-degree angle with your body. If need be, prop your feet on a footstool or large book to help achieve this.
- Lay your baby on his side so that you are 'tummy to tummy'. If it helps, use a pillow across your lap to support your baby and bring him in line with your breast.
- Pull your baby closer to your breast and support his neck and shoulders with the hand that is by his feet. It is very important to

support his head by having your arm come up his back, with your thumb and fingers gently curling round his neck rather than actually holding the back of his head. This is because he can feel restricted by having pressure on the back of his head – he will be unable to move his head freely and it tends to push his chin towards his chest (see next point).

○ To be able to swallow easily, your baby's head needs to be slightly tilted back to open up his throat and allow for maximum jaw movement. If you try swallowing with your chin tucked into your chest and then with your head tilted slightly back, you will experience for yourself how difficult it is for your baby to swallow if his head is pushed forward towards his chest.

○ With your free hand – i.e. the hand by your baby's head – support your breast and gently squeeze it so that your nipple is pushed slightly forwards.

○ Bring your baby towards your breast and brush his mouth and cheeks around your nipple.

○ It can be useful to squeeze out a few drops of milk to encourage your baby's 'rooting' reflex.

○ Watch for your baby to open his mouth, hopefully nice and wide, and pull him quickly towards your breast and on to your nipple.

○ Always pull your baby towards your breast rather than leaning forwards and trying to push your breast into his mouth.

○ As he begins to suck, the initial, toe-curling pain should quickly pass as he draws the nipple towards the back of his throat and his tongue works on the areola by pushing and releasing it against the roof of his mouth. This puts on–off pressure on the ducts lying behind the areola and forces the milk to move out of them and squirt through the nipple.

○ If it is really sore and the pain doesn't pass after a minute or two, take him off and adjust your position slightly, then try again.

○ To break the latch, ease your little finger into his mouth and gently prise his mouth off your nipple.

○ The sign of a good latch is when his lips are curled outwards and a large amount of areola is drawn into his mouth.

○ Ensure that he is able to breathe freely and his nostrils are not blocked by or squashed into your breast tissue.

○ Once he is comfortably latched on, relax the hand supporting your breast and make sure you are not blocking the milk flow with your fingers.

○ You may be able to remove the hand that is supporting him if he is comfortable and supported on a pillow.

○ Watch for the whole of your baby's jaw to be rhythmically moving. He should fall into a pattern of sucking for a couple of minutes and then resting while still latched on.

○ Although you need to concentrate on how your baby is feeding and it is tempting to want to gaze adoringly at him all the time, be careful not to look down continually as it can cause you to get a really stiff neck.

○ You should also be able to hear a pattern of contented swallowing and breathing noises if he is drinking efficiently.

○ If he stops sucking for more than a few minutes, gently encourage him to carry on by stroking his cheek, tickling his chin or feet, or gently blowing on his face.

○ If it is fairly warm or you find your baby is often quite sleepy, then you may need to undress him before a feed to wake him up.

○ Being 'skin to skin' will often encourage your baby to feed more efficiently.

How long and which breast?

Again, this is completely individual to each mum and baby, but, based on experience, to help establish and maintain your milk supply I would advise the following:

○ Become 'breast aware'. Before feeding, feel your breasts; then do it again after the feed. This can help give you some confidence that your baby has had a good feed, as your breasts will feel softer and less heavy after feeding than they did before you started.

○ At each feed offer the first breast for around 20 minutes. The time actually spent at the first breast can vary from as little as 15 to as much as 45 minutes, but I believe that generally most babies will take pretty much what they need within the first 20 minutes of a feed and will also be most easily able to obtain milk within this time.

○ Offer the second breast when you feel that the first has been emptied. Some babies may not want to take the second breast, but even if they latch on and suck for only a few minutes it does help to stimulate your supply.

○ My guideline is usually 20–45 minutes for the first breast and 5–20 minutes for the second. This also helps to keep each feed to within an hour, otherwise each one seems to roll into the next.

○ Begin each feed by offering the breast that you fed from last at the previous feed. Many mums struggle to remember which breast they last fed from, so keeping a chart can be a help (see the sample chart on page 114 and also 'Your Journal' on page 253).

○ The timing of a feed is from when you started, not from when it ended. So if one started at 10.30am, no matter how long it took the next feed would be due around 1.30pm.

○ If your baby is sleepy after feeding at the first breast, then try a nappy change to wake him up before offering the other.

○ If your baby is simply not interested, or is too sleepy to feed, put him down and try again in half an hour or so. This may mean you need to adapt your feeding plan slightly so that you can still end up with bedtime at around 7pm.

○ Do remember that each breastfeed will be different from the last. They will take varying amounts of time, some will go well, some may be disasters, some will fall nicely into the 3-hour feeding plan while others may seem to be completely random . . . but don't panic, persevere for as long as you feel comfortable and if you want to offer a bottle of either expressed milk or formula instead to give yourself a break, then do so – there is no need to feel guilty!

Expressing breast milk

It is possible to express your breasts manually and many mums will find it useful to learn how to do this, firstly to encourage a newborn to suckle by producing a few drops of breast milk which will stimulate the baby's sense of smell and taste, and secondly because if their breasts become slightly engorged the nipples can flatten out, making it harder for the baby to latch on. Manually expressing a small amount of breast milk before the feed will make the breast slightly softer, allowing the baby to get a better latch. Stretch out your thumb and forefingers and, using the flat of your hand, apply gentle pressure in a downward motion from the base of your breast towards the nipple. Repeat this motion a few times and the milk should soon start to flow. If you are going to express more than a few drops do make sure to use a sterile bowl in which to catch the milk.

You may be told that a breast pump is not as efficient as your baby and that pumping will have a detrimental effect on your milk production, but I do not believe this to be the case. In fact, even though the use of a breast pump may not stimulate the high levels of the hormone prolactin that is found in a mother whose baby feeds at the breast, it can still sustain an entirely satisfactory milk supply. This is proved, for example, by the many mothers whose babies are in special care units, and so cannot be put to the breast to feed, who can still provide the necessary milk – and often more than is needed – by the regular use of a breast pump. Also, I have worked with many other mums who, for one reason or another, choose not to put their baby to the breast at all but prefer to express all their milk and give it through a bottle. Some have even sustained this for well over six months, thus disproving the theory that expressing can be detrimental to your milk production and supply.

There are many different pumps on the market and unfortunately it is often only after you have bought one and tried it out that you discover whether it is the model that is best suited to you. In my experience the mini electric pumps are probably the best and tend to suit most women. It is possible to hire breast pumps from your local branch of the National Childbirth Trust (NCT) or from a hospital on a weekly or monthly basis; your midwife or health visitor should be able to give you more information on this.

Again, expressing is a totally individual experience: some mums hate it and others use it as their preferred feeding method, as mentioned above.

If you have chosen exclusively to use breast milk for your baby, then it is advisable to try to get to grips with expressing some milk at least once or twice a day. This milk can then be used to replace one breastfeed during the night, or used as top-ups at feeds towards the end of a busy and tiring day as your supply naturally diminishes. It will also introduce your baby to a bottle in the first couple of weeks which will help to avoid rejection of the bottle at a later stage.

Some mums find expressing relatively easy and can pump off 90ml in 10 minutes or so, while others can take half an hour just to get 20ml. If you find that you don't like or don't get on with pumping but still want to substitute a couple of feeds, then obviously you can use formula.

When to express?

I usually advise expressing first thing in the morning, straight after the first feed. Your milk should be in reasonable supply as you have rested throughout the night and more often than not you will have more than your baby needs for this first feed of the day. Then express again just before going to bed and supplement the first night feed with a bottle – perhaps your partner will be able to give this feed so you can get some rest.

The following chart gives an example of when to feed and when to express and suggests feed times for a fully breastfed, full-term baby on Days 16 and 17. A supply of expressed milk has already been built up, as expressing started on Day 6. If you have substituted the previous feed and expressed both breasts or expressed after giving the last feed, it doesn't really matter which breast you start with for the next.

L = left breast, R = right breast.

Example of when to feed and when to express

6.30am	Breastfeed: L 35 mins, R 10 mins
7.30am	Express both breasts: 85ml
9.45am	Breastfeed: R 45 mins, L 20 mins
1pm	Breastfeed: L 25 mins, R 15 mins
4pm	Breastfeed: R 40 mins, L 15 mins
5.15pm	Obviously hungry so gave expressed top-up of 40ml

6.45pm	Breastfeed: L 20 mins, R 20 mins; expressed top-up of 30ml
9.30pm	Expressed 140ml
12.30am	Expressed feed with daddy: 140ml
4.30am	Breastfeed: R 30 mins; didn't offer other side
7.30am	Breastfeed: L 25 mins, R 10 mins
8.15am	Expressed 120ml
10.30am	Breastfeed: R 20 mins, L 15 mins
11.15am	Had a spare 10 mins so expressed again: 60ml
1.40pm	Breastfeed: L 35 mins, R 20 mins
4.20pm	Breastfeed: R 45 mins, L 15 mins
6.50pm	Breastfeed: L 20 mins, R 20 mins; expressed top-up of 70ml
9.10pm	Expressed 150ml
1.30am	Expressed feed: 160ml
5am	Breastfeed: L 15 mins; baby fell asleep so put back to bed to try to stay on track for morning feed
7.15am	Breastfeed: R 30 mins, L 15 mins
8.15am	Expressed 130ml
	And so on . . .

Storage

Before expressing, all the pump equipment and storage bottles should be washed and sterilized. If freezing breast milk, storage bags are very useful. Breast milk can safely be stored in a fridge for up to 48 hours (although some do say for longer), but my advice is to freeze your breast milk straight away unless you know you are going to use it within the next day or two. It can be stored for up to six months in a proper freezer or up to three months in the freezer compartment of a fridge. Thaw it by leaving it for a few hours at room temperature or by standing it in a jug of hot water to defrost more quickly. Once milk has been defrosted it should not be re-frozen, and once warmed for use it should be used within an hour or so and any leftover milk should be thrown away. Breast milk can be warmed the same as any other milk, either by standing it in a jug of hot water or using a bottle-warmer.

Temporary substitution for breast milk

Expressing can be useful if you need to take prescribed medications like antibiotics while you are breastfeeding. Although many health professionals and doctors advise that it is safe to take antibiotics while breastfeeding, I am not so sure as I have observed a link between the onset of digestive issues in some breastfed babies and their mums taking certain antibiotics. My advice is to read the antibiotic information leaflet and if it lists heartburn or gastric discomfort as side-effects in the patient, then you can assume that this might cause similar problems in the baby. I would suggest that you 'pump and dump' while taking the medication, feeding your baby either stored expressed milk and/or formula and resuming breastfeeding once you have finished taking the course of tablets. I will be completely honest here: it may be that your baby will not re-accept the breast after getting used to a bottle for a number of days and you may then have to give up breastfeeding or continue to pump and give him expressed milk. Some mothers, however, have found that although it has taken a difficult couple of days, after much perseverance they do successfully get their baby to breastfeed again.

Expressing also gives you the option of a more flexible feeding pattern, as you can pump and leave milk for someone else to feed your baby. To maintain your supply, though, it is important to try to pump at the time that you should have been feeding. However, if you do just miss the odd feed here and there and don't pump instead, it really should be OK.

So if for any reason you are going to pump for a few days and then hope to resume breastfeeding, you will need to express roughly at the same times, or at least for the same number of times each day, that you would normally put your baby to the breast.

Reducing your milk supply to give up breastfeeding

When the time comes that you decide to stop breastfeeding, you will need to think about how quickly or slowly you want to achieve this. Ideally it will be a gradual withdrawal over a number of weeks, which gives your body the chance to re-adjust. If you give up too quickly, your breasts will become engorged, which is extremely painful. However, there are many different reasons why a mum may decide to give up breastfeeding and many different ways and time scales in which to accomplish it. The following examples give advice on the most common experiences.

Deciding not to breastfeed from birth

If you have decided not to breastfeed, although your mind knows your decision your body hasn't quite yet got the message and directly after the birth your hormones will spring into action and start the whole milk-production process. Your milk will still 'come in' at the usual time, even though you may not have put your baby to the breast at all. However, it is usually fairly shortlived if your breasts are not stimulated by your baby sucking. Although you may experience some engorgement and discomfort for a few days, painkillers will help and your milk should quite quickly disappear. Your breasts will return to normal within a week or so.

Giving up all at once

I call this 'going cold turkey'. Although it is the quickest route to giving up breastfeeding, it can be the most painful. Years ago doctors would prescribe a drug, such as Bromocriptine, to help 'dry up' the milk, but it is not common practice through the NHS today so you will need to go it alone. Arm yourself with paracetamol and ibuprofen tablets and take the maximum prescribed dose for three or four days immediately after you give up. Cold compresses applied to the breasts can help relieve the pain and warm showers or hot baths can also help by letting some of the milk flow out to relieve the pressure rather than expressing the milk, which continues to stimulate the supply.

For women who decide to give up this way it can be a very painful three or four days before the milk starts to disappear – woe betide anyone who gets too near and accidentally knocks their boobs! You will also need to be careful that you don't get a bout of mastitis. Check your breasts three or four times each day and if you find a hot, red, hard lump starting to form, try getting in the bath or under the shower and gently massaging the area around the lump with your fingers or thumbs, stroking it away towards the nipple. If it doesn't disappear or if you start to feel any flu-like symptoms, then you should seek medical advice straight away. See also page 57.

Giving up straight away but reducing your supply by expressing

If you have decided to give up putting your baby to the breast but are happy to express for a little while longer, then this is probably an easier option than going cold turkey. You can make gradual reductions to the quantity and the number of times that you pump until your milk has all but disappeared, which will usually take ten to fourteen days for an established milk supply. If you have still been breastfeeding at night, then I suggest it is better not to replace the nighttime feeds with pumping – express only during the day and before going to bed. Try to put a 4-hourly schedule of expressing in place, for instance at 8am, noon, 4pm and 8pm – but if you do need to express a little bit in between times, then do so. However, do remember that each time you express you are still stimulating your breasts to produce more milk, so the less pumping you have to do the better. Over a number of days you will need to reduce the amount you pump and cut back on the time it takes to express so that by around Day 3 or 4 you should be down to pumping just three times a day. Some women find that their breast milk dries up fairly quickly, whereas for others it can take up to two weeks or so and you will need to reduce your expressing accordingly.

Giving up by gradually removing breastfeeds

If you want to give up by gradually weaning your baby off the breast, then the following tables will give you an idea of how best to achieve this. They are only examples and you may find you need to adapt the schedule to suit you and your baby, maybe expressing here and there in place of feeding. For instance, you may decide to offer the breast at bedtime and top up with a bottlefeed for a longer period of time, or you may decide to give up that breastfeed straight away, which means you will need to express before going to bed so that you are not too uncomfortable during the night.

Example 1: A 4-week-old baby

Day	7am	10am	1pm	4pm	7pm	12am	4am
1	breast	breast	breast	breast	breast	bottle	bottle
2	breast	breast	breast	breast	breast	bottle	bottle
3	breast	breast	bottle	breast	breast	bottle	bottle
4	breast	breast	bottle	breast	small breast with bottle top-up	2am bottle	
5	breast	breast	bottle	breast	small breast with bottle top-up	"	"

Day	7am	10am	1pm	4pm	7pm	12am	4am
6	breast	breast	bottle	breast	bottle	2am bottle	
7	breast	breast	bottle	breast	bottle	"	"
8	breast	bottle	bottle	breast	bottle	3am bottle	
9	breast	bottle	bottle	breast	bottle	"	"
10	breast	bottle	bottle	breast	bottle	"	"
11	breast	bottle	bottle	breast	bottle	"	"
12	breast	bottle	bottle	breast	bottle	4am bottle	
13	breast	bottle	bottle	bottle	bottle	"	"
14	bottle	bottle	bottle	bottle	bottle	"	"

Example 2: An 8-week-old baby

Day	7am	10am	1pm	4pm	7pm
1	breast	breast	breast	breast	breast
2	breast	breast	breast	breast	breast
3	breast	breast	bottle	breast	breast
4	breast	breast	bottle	breast	small breast with bottle top-up
5	breast	breast	bottle	breast	small breast with bottle top-up

Day	7am	10am	1pm	4pm	7pm
6	breast	breast	bottle	breast	bottle
7	breast	breast	bottle	breast	bottle
8	breast	bottle	bottle	breast	bottle
9	breast	bottle	bottle	breast	bottle
10	breast	bottle	bottle	breast	bottle
11	breast	bottle	bottle	breast	bottle
12	breast	bottle	bottle	breast	bottle
13	breast	bottle	bottle	bottle	bottle
14	bottle	bottle	bottle	bottle	bottle

Example 3: A 16-week-old baby

Day	7am	11am	2.30pm	6.30pm
1	breast	bottle	breast	breast
2	breast	bottle	breast	breast
3	breast	bottle	breast	breast
4	breast	bottle	breast	bottle
5	breast	bottle	breast	bottle
6	breast	bottle	breast	bottle

Day	7am	11am	2.30pm	6.30pm
7	breast	bottle	breast	bottle
8	breast	bottle	breast	bottle
9	breast	bottle	bottle	bottle
10	breast	bottle	bottle	bottle
11	breast	bottle	bottle	bottle
12	breast	bottle	bottle	bottle
13	breast	bottle	bottle	bottle
14	bottle	bottle	bottle	bottle

Breastfeeding problems

Sadly, breastfeeding is not always straightforward. Some of the most common difficulties are explained below.

Sore and cracked nipples

Undoubtedly the main cause of sore or damaged nipples is incorrect positioning of your baby at the breast. As with most things, prevention is better than cure and by following my advice on a feeding schedule as set out in this plan, as well as my guidelines on positioning and the latch (see pages 40–43), then I hope you will avoid too many problems. Even though you follow this advice, however, it is still possible for problems to occur because of certain factors beyond your control:

○ If you have had a Caesarean section it may mean that you cannot move about easily and this can make it difficult to get into a comfortable position, with the knock-on effect of not getting the baby's position or latch spot on in the first few days after giving birth.

○ Some babies are born with a tongue-tie and this, nearly always, will cause difficulty in breastfeeding. A tongue-tie occurs when the cord (or frenum) underneath the tongue is attached too far down towards the tip of the tongue, restricting its movement. This means that the baby will not be able to draw into his mouth enough of the surrounding areola and will only be able to suck on the nipple itself, which will soon make it extremely sore. The cord will need to be snipped (a frenotomy) and this should be done as soon as possible after birth. Some midwives specialize in carrying out this procedure and many hospitals have a 'tongue-tie clinic' once a week. If it is left uncut for too long it will be necessary for the baby to have a general anaesthetic to rectify the problem.

○ Some babies are born with a reflux problem and therefore have issues with feeding, which may prevent them from latching-on or sucking at the breast properly. This will result in extremely sore nipples. See Chapter 6 on dealing with reflux and feeding problems.

If you do find your nipples get sore, there are a number of things that might help. Different methods work for different individuals, so try some of the following tips to find what suits you best:

○ Avoid washing your breasts with soap too often as this can take away the natural oils and cause the nipples to dry out and crack.

○ Rubbing a few drops of breast milk on to and around the nipple after each feed can help.

○ There are a multitude of creams, potions and lotions on the market. Quite simply, some mums find they help and some don't. During my survey I have found that Lasinoh cream seems to be favoured by most. Some professionals advise that creams should be avoided, but if you find one that helps then use it!

○ Many mums find that nipple shields work really well by protecting sore nipples during a feed. They are made from a soft, pliable latex-type material that comfortably fits over your nipple and the surrounding areola, giving the baby a larger and more defined teat on which to latch. Again, though, their use is frowned upon by some breastfeeding advisers, as they believe they will only encourage the baby to suck on an artificial teat instead of breastfeeding in the 'proper' way. My advice is to try them if and when necessary, and continue with their use if it helps.

○ If a nipple has become extremely sore and cracked, it may be necessary to 'rest' that particular breast by expressing for the next few feeds. Nipples can become sore very quickly, but when rested will usually heal very quickly too.

Blocked ducts

A blocked duct can occur at any time throughout lactation, restricting the flow of milk through the breast and into the nipple. The milk then accumulates behind the blockage and may become noticeable as a hard, knobbly lump which may be painful. Sometimes there seems to be no reason for this occurring, but in general the most probable causes are:

○ The breast not being adequately emptied at each feed.
○ Not being able to achieve a comfortable position for your baby, resulting in an incorrect latch.
○ The pressure of an incorrectly fitting bra.
○ An accidental knock or blow to a breast that causes some bruising.
○ Allowing your baby to feed too frequently at the breast, which results in the hind-milk not being drained off and the milk fat then blocking the duct.

Prevention:
○ Ensure that your baby is always correctly positioned at the breast and that the latch is as good as you can get it (see pages 40–43).
○ If your baby is struggling with breastfeeding, still put him to the breast to encourage him but then express the breasts after each feed.
○ Try another feeding position, such as the 'rugby-ball' technique. This is when you tuck your baby under your arm with his head to the breast and his feet down your side, as opposed to laying him across your tummy.

Treatment:

○ Start the next feed on the affected side in the hope that a hungry baby's vigorous sucking will clear the blockage.

○ Gently massage the lump towards the nipple with your free hand while your baby is feeding.

○ Apply a warm flannel or heat pad to the affected area to help the milk flow.

○ Fully express the breasts after each feed.

Mastitis

This can occur as the result of a blocked duct being unnoticed and left untreated. The lump that originally formed from the blocked duct will grow in size and become red, sore, hot and inflamed, which usually indicates that there is an infection lurking within the affected area. You may have a temperature, feel cold and shivery, and show general flu-like symptoms.

Treatment:

○ Feed your baby for as often and as long as he wants. This will keep the breast milk flowing, which is often the root of the problem. Gently massage any lumpy or blocked areas while baby is feeding.

○ Always try to ensure correct positioning.

○ Express milk as often as possible.

○ Try to rest and increase your fluid intake.

○ Some professionals advise to continue breastfeeding at all costs, but I believe it is up to the individual to make her own decision and if you do not feel comfortable with putting your baby to the breast then substitute bottlefeeds, ensuring that you express instead.

○ Putting a cold compress on the affected area may help.

○ Pain relief, as directed by a doctor.

○ If the symptoms do not subside after a few hours, then you should seek medical advice. It may mean that you will need a course of antibiotics to clear up the infection. For my advice on this, see page 48.

Breast abscess

Delayed treatment of mastitis may result in the formation of a breast abscess. It is a fairly rare condition but will need immediate medical attention. Rigorous pumping and hot and cold compresses, along with antibiotics, may be enough to treat the abscess if it is diagnosed relatively early on. At its worst there may be blood and pus oozing from the nipple and you will feel extremely unwell with severe flu-like symptoms. Treatment often entails a surgical procedure to drain the infected area.

White spots

Sometimes small white spots appear on the tips of the nipples. This can mean that the openings of the milk ducts on to the nipples are blocked with an accumulation of milk solids. Very occasionally, a thin layer of skin may grow over the openings on the nipple, making them look like tiny, milk-filled blisters. If this occurs and does not improve with feeding or expression, the 'blisters' may have to be punctured with a sterile needle.

Thrush

This is a very painful condition that can develop either on the mother's nipples or as oral thrush in the baby's mouth. If you are susceptible to bouts of vaginal thrush then there is an increased chance of it occurring on your nipples when you breastfeed. More commonly it is caused by either you or your baby having to take a course of antibiotics.

On the breasts there may be tiny, white, itchy spots on or around the nipples which become extremely sore during and after feeding. You may experience shooting pains through your breasts and it may even feel like red hot needles being driven into your breasts. If your baby gets oral thrush, then his mouth and tongue will become covered in definite white spots and will have a general white coating that cannot be wiped off with a clean finger. Thrush does need medical treatment and both you and your baby should be prescribed an anti-fungal medication.

Inverted or flat nipples

It is simply not the case that, no matter what size or shape your nipples, your baby is designed to fit them perfectly. Flat or inverted nipples can cause huge problems when trying to get your baby to latch on. Ignore weird and wonderful suggestions such as using a syringe to help 'pull out' and stretch your nipples: the best and easiest solution is to use nipple shields. You may always have to use them, or perhaps as your baby grows he may get strong enough to latch on without them.

Mum's the Word . . .

When Louis was born he was a big, 9lb baby. I watched him lose weight until he was only 7.5lb at four weeks old. I was only advised by my health visitor when he was five weeks old to start him on formula. When I did this he had been breastfeeding every couple of hours and both he and I were in a terrible state.

The advice Alison gave me was simple, really easy to follow, did not require me to write anything complicated down and also allowed me to enjoy my time with my new little boy. In a few weeks he was a different baby. He gained nearly a pound each week and was sleeping through at ten weeks.

A. R.

Bottle- and formula-feeding

It is a shame in today's society that formula-feeding, when used in preference to breastfeeding, is almost frowned upon – to the point of making some women feel that they are 'bad mothers' if they choose it rather than breastfeeding. The first formulas designed to replace breast milk were produced commercially in 1867 and were used to remove the need for the wet nurse and also to save the lives of those babies whose mothers had either died, could not produce any milk or were unable to breastfeed. Since its introduction all those years ago, formula has continued to improve in quality and most types now even contain lipids and pro-biotics, making them more similar to breast milk than ever before. Most babies will thrive and easily accept the usual dairy formulas which are readily available, although some who suffer intolerances, allergies or gastro-oesophageal reflux will do better with one of the many specialized formulas; see Chapter 7.

> ### *Alison says . . .*
>
> I often wonder if human breast milk is the 'natural' food it is always claimed to be these days. If you stop to consider the 'unnatural' methods used in the production of the foods we eat – genetic modification, over-cultivation, pest control and animal management – how can we be sure that our breast milk remains 'pure' and unaffected?

A recent article in *The Times* suggests that much of the recent research promoting breastfeeding over formula is actually flawed.[5] The article highlights the fact that statistics cannot truly prove that breastfed children have higher IQs than those fed on formula, as there are too many other contributing factors that are not taken into account. The main fact is that the majority of babies who are fed with breast milk are known to be born to parents in the middle to upper classes and their children will probably enjoy a higher standard of education. So although the majority of breastfed babies may prove to have better outcomes in life, this could easily be due to factors that were not taken into account when the statistics were compiled.

Bonding with your baby

Many breastfeeding advisers say that it is more difficult to bond with your baby if you don't breastfeed, but in my experience this is simply not true. A mum who has chosen to bottlefeed from the start will not know anything different and will build up a bond with her baby the same as any mother who breastfeeds. Also, any mum who switches to bottlefeeding after a not-so-happy breastfeeding experience will probably find it to be far more positively bonding and a lot less stressful for both herself and the baby.

It is a strange fact that 'bonding with your baby' is often mentioned only with regard to feeding. I believe that a large part of the bonding process takes place at other times too. Also, in my experience it can sometimes be easier to build a bond through being able to maintain eye contact while holding your baby in a bottlefeeding position.

How to hold your baby while bottlefeeding

You might be surprised to find that I actually have anything to write about a position for a bottlefeed! Surely positioning is all about breastfeeding? Well, I have found this to be an important yet very little talked-about topic, and one that can have a major effect on your baby's ability to feed well.

It seems to be a natural instinct to cradle your baby close to your body, nestled in the crook of your arm, when giving a bottlefeed, but this position can actually create an unnatural 'kink' in your baby's digestive tract, making it more difficult for the milk to flow to his stomach. Whether breast- or bottlefeeding, the baby's body needs to be kept as straight as possible to allow the milk to flow freely down his oesophagus and into his stomach. Also, when a baby is held in the crook of an arm, it can cause his head to tilt forwards so that his chin is tucked into his chest, making it more difficult for him to suck and swallow. If anything, a baby's head needs to be tilted slightly backwards to allow for full movement of his jaw while he sucks and the free passage of milk down his throat.

You will need to experiment to find a feeding position that suits both you and your baby. Very often a pillow or cushion placed across your lap can help support him while keeping him in the prone position.

Bottles and teats

There are so many different makes on the market today that it must seem like a complete minefield when trying to choose which brand to use. For ease of use, my personal preferences are the basic Avent bottles, along with either a steam or microwave sterilizer.

There are many makes of bottle that claim to 'reduce wind', are 'anti-colic' and some that claim to be just like a breast – but I truly have not found any of these claims to be substantiated and many of these complicated bottles just create more bits and pieces to wash up and sterilize, making what is a tedious task at the best of times even longer.

Undoubtedly there are some instances where specialized bottles and/or teats may be necessary. For instance, premature babies, those with cleft palates or any that have severe feeding problems may not be able to suck efficiently from an ordinary bottle. Softer, smaller and more pliable teats may help.

Whatever bottles you choose, do always check that you are using teats with a hole size that matches your baby's ability to suck. Nearly all teats are sold in age ranges, but many babies need a larger-holed teat sooner than the age recommendation states. If the teat is too small then it may cause the baby to gulp and suck too hard, which in turn can lead to problems with excessive wind. It is really trial and error to find which teat size suits your baby at any particular age. If you think he needs to move up a size because feeds seem to be taking longer and longer, then just try it out. You will soon be able to tell if the flow is too fast, as he may well cough, splutter or gag on the milk if too much is getting through.

Alison says . . .

There has been much in the press lately about bottles containing Bisphenol A (BPA), a chemical used in plastics, and so being unsafe. I suggest you carry out your own research on this. However, many brands are now being made as BPA-free.

Making up and storing bottles

Each brand and make of formula comes with its own instructions for use. There are also new guidelines in place with regard to making up feeds, as there is some concern that, once opened, a box of milk powder is then not sterile and should be added to very hot water to kill any bacteria. It is important to read and follow the manufacturers' guidelines on preparing feeds, but I have found the easiest and most practical way – which is still, in my opinion, safe – to prepare and store bottles is as follows:

○ Wash, rinse and sterilize all the bottles and teats.
○ Boil some fresh water in a clean kettle and leave it to cool for 10 to 15 minutes.
○ Add the required amount of water to each bottle and seal it by putting on the assembled screw-on neck, teat and cap.
○ Store the bottles in a fridge or leave them in a safe place on the worktop or in a cupboard.
○ As feed time approaches, add the appropriate amount of formula to one bottle, mix it thoroughly by shaking and then warm as required. Some babies seem to like having their feed at room temperature, whereas others prefer it to be fairly warm.
○ I suggest that you have enough bottles that you need only wash, sterilize and prepare the water once a day and add the formula at each feed time.
○ If your baby initially refuses his feed, you can re-offer the same bottle up to an hour later. After that the feed should be discarded and a fresh one made up.

Making up and storing bottles in this way is also the easiest way to give bottle feeds when out and about and travelling. You can measure out the required scoops of formula into a suitable, clean plastic container (these are readily available on the market as formula dispensers) to take with you along with your pre-prepared bottle of water and add when you are ready to feed.

☆ *Alison's Golden Rules* ☆

1   Choose, without feeling pressurized, the method of feeding that is best for you and your baby.

2   Remember, breastfeeding is an art that needs to be learned by both you and your baby. It doesn't necessarily come naturally.

3   When breastfeeding, if you want the flexibility of ever using a bottle within your feeding schedule, then you must introduce and keep in place at least one bottlefeed every day during the first two weeks.

4   Whether breast- or bottlefeeding, make sure that you position your baby so that his head is tilted slightly backwards and his chin is not tucked into his chest.

5   Where possible, try to stick to your 3-hourly feeding plan and wake your baby for feeds during the day if necessary.

6   Persevere with feeds during the day to ensure that your baby takes enough milk to help him get through the night.

7   Never continually 'force' your baby to take a feed. If he is not ready, wait, try again a little later and adjust the rest of the day accordingly.

8   If you are struggling with feeding in any way, seek help and don't be fobbed off until you are happy that things are improving.

9   Keep a diary of feeds and times for the first few weeks: it will be useful to refer back to it if problems should occur.

10   If you choose at any point to use formula to feed your baby – don't feel guilty.

3

All About Sleep

Sleep is a naturally occurring fact of life which nearly all creatures in the animal kingdom need to survive. The rest that it gives is the mainstay of the body's growth and rejuvenation and without it we would not be able to live.

Why then has it become such a complicated, problematical and misunderstood part of our lives? Why is it often dismissed and neglected as being trivial and unimportant? This is especially true when a new baby arrives in your family. The idea that you are going to undergo months and even years of sleepless and disturbed nights seems to be accepted as the norm and you are expected, somehow, to 'just cope'!

Basically, most babies are born nocturnal and it is very important to re-train them within the first few weeks of life. When a baby is in the womb he is often lulled and rocked to sleep during the day by his mother's movements as she goes about her normal daytime activities. When she lies down in bed at night to rest he has more room to move about, and without the comfort of motion he will often become more wakeful. Recognizing the associations with sleep and the nocturnal pattern that evolves in the womb should make us realize that babies need to learn new and independent methods of settling themselves to sleep which will fit into their new 'outside' world of night and day.

Let's start at the beginning: night and day

Through following this plan you will learn how to re-educate your baby's sleep habits during his first few weeks of life. The following points will help you when trying to establish the important difference between night and day:

○ Ensure that the nursery is reasonably dark throughout the night. It is not necessary to use actual blackout blinds; most ordinary curtains or blinds will suffice. Remember, babies learn by association, so if they are used only to complete darkness a change of environment – to a hotel room, for instance – where more light gets in may cause problems when trying to get them to sleep.

○ When your baby has woken and you are ready to get him up, open the curtains in his room to indicate that it is morning and time to start the day before you get him out of his cot.

○ Whether it is before or after the first feed, at some point give your baby his morning wash and change him out of his night wear into fresh, daytime clothes. This can be as simple as using all-in-one suits and keeping white for night and coloured for day.

○ It is important that your baby is able to take enough food during the day to enable him to sleep for longer at night, so always wake him during the day to stay roughly on schedule for his daytime feeds.

Alison says . . .

In my opinion you should never have to wake a sleeping baby at night for a feed, unless there is a medical reason to do so.

○ Follow a set sequence for feeds and nap times during the day, then aim towards an early-evening bathtime, which will become the focal part of establishing a good bedtime routine. As your baby gets older, you will find that the bedtime routine you have put in place from the start will continue for years to come to encourage a healthy association with going to bed and then to sleep.

Alison says . . .

I do appreciate that a calm, peaceful bedtime routine is much easier to achieve with your first baby. When you have a lively toddler to cope with or an older child who needs your attention, bedtime can become a really difficult time of day to manage. See Chapter 4 for advice on how to deal with this.

○   Where possible, the last feed of the day, which from now on I shall refer to as 'the bedtime feed', should be carried out in a calm, quiet atmosphere. I suggest you use the room in which your baby is going to go to bed, dim the lights and try to keep things as relaxed as possible.

○   Resist the temptation to fill your baby's cot with stimulating toys and mobiles. This is his bed and should therefore be a calm, peaceful place in which to sleep.

○   In the early weeks when night feeds are still necessary, keep the bedroom lights as low as possible, don't overstimulate your baby and try to carry out the whole process with a minimum of fuss. It has been said that when doing night feeds you should not talk to or look at your baby at all, but he will feel more reassured by some loving words spoken in a calm, quiet voice.

Encouraging a positive association with sleep

As I have already mentioned, an important part of encouraging good sleep habits in your baby is to help him discover his own way of settling himself to sleep. This becomes one of the fundamental steps in encouraging him to sleep through the night. When it is time either for a nap or for bedtime, it is important for your baby to be aware and awake enough to realize that he has been put into his cot. This helps to form the association of going into his cot awake and then settling himself to sleep without any assistance. He needs to become familiar with his sleeping area and bedtime surroundings so that he feels comfortable, safe and relaxed when drifting off to sleep.

In the early weeks you may find it difficult to put your baby into his cot while he is still awake as the temptation is often to let him fall asleep while you are feeding, holding or cuddling him. Of course it is fine to let him fall asleep in this way occasionally, and you will both enjoy the closeness it can bring, but do try to resist the temptation to let it become a habit, as your baby may then decide that he *only* wants to sleep this way. For example, as most sleep times follow a feed, it may seem easier with a very young baby who has dozed off while feeding to put him into his cot already asleep, as it seems unkind to wake him. However, although your baby may be quite sleepy after his feed, my advice is to move him gently and stimulate him so that he stirs and becomes aware that you are putting him into his cot. Transferring him to his cot without waking him at all will only leave him with the association of falling asleep while being fed and he will quickly come to rely on feeding to help him go to sleep. This may then lead to your baby insisting on frequent nighttime feeds, as when he wakes or stirs through his sleep cycles and realizes he is not at the breast or being fed he will not want to re-settle himself without the comfort of feeding to which he has become accustomed.

Mum's the Word . . .

We were so thrilled with our beautiful baby girl that during the early weeks we found it was really hard ever to put her down and loved feeling so close to her as she slept in our arms. But little did we realize the rod we had made for our own backs! By Week 3 our baby would not sleep anywhere unless she was being cuddled and this was throughout the night too – we were soon exhausted.

Alison showed us how to re-train her by constant re-settling and reassurance when putting her into her cot. Luckily, within three days she had accepted her cot and was 'sleeping like a baby'!

J. T.

Following this same pattern, your baby can easily become reliant on other types of sleep aid that you may have introduced while trying to get him to settle. The most common things that babies learn to rely on for sleep are:

○ a dummy
○ being rocked, patted or shushed to sleep
○ movement – for instance, being in a pram, car or swing seat

○ listening to music or 'white noise'
○ watching a mobile
○ being caressed or having their hand held

Again, the issue with your baby becoming used to one or more of these sleep aids is that very quickly he will be unable to fall asleep without it. For instance, he may happily drift off to sleep while you sit next to him stroking his head and holding his hand, but then when he wakes or stirs during his sleep cycles the last thing he will remember about going to sleep is your comforting caress, so he may not be able to re-settle himself to sleep without it. As a result, in addition to feed times you could also be up and down all night long having to comfort him back to sleep!

Settling your baby to sleep

I do realize that settling your baby to sleep may sometimes be quite tricky, but on the whole, as long as he is feeding well most of the time, he should usually be able to settle to sleep fairly easily. If he is struggling to settle it may be for one of these reasons:

○ He may still be hungry.
○ He may have wind.
○ He may be too hot or, rarely, too cold.
○ He may have a dirty nappy.
○ He may have abdominal discomfort leading to a bowel movement.
○ He may be overtired and therefore irritable and unable to settle.
○ He may be uncomfortable if he is on his back and being disturbed by his 'startle reflex' (see pages 73–4).
○ He may have digestive issues causing acid reflux and heartburn-like pain when he lies down (see Chapter 7).
○ He may be feeling unwell.

When you put your baby down for a nap or at bedtime and he doesn't go to sleep straight away, instead of tending to him immediately try to leave him for 5–10 minutes or so to see if he is going to settle down or not. If you then decide that he needs attention due to one of the reasons mentioned above, then it should be fairly simple to offer more feed, change him, wind him or make sure that he is comfortable and then re-settle him back into the cot for his sleep. To help you understand what may be preventing your baby from going to sleep, look back over the last few feeds, sleeps and nappy changes and you may be able to work out the cause fairly easily. For instance, if he hasn't had a dirty nappy for a few hours a good guess might be that he is building up for a big poo. You may find it useful to compile a simple chart or diary similar to the example on pages 113–14 to help keep track of what happened when.

If your baby continually struggles to settle and you find it almost impossible to get him to go into his cot for a sleep, then you need to look at other possible causes. Any signs of illness or high temperatures, etc., will need to be discussed and investigated by your GP. One major cause of a baby being reluctant or unable to settle easily can be traced to the medical condition reflux, but unfortunately this is rarely diagnosed in the early weeks. A baby with this condition can suffer from severe heartburn-like pain, especially when lying flat on his back, and it may cause him to cry or even scream as soon as he is put down. It may also trigger a fit of crying as soon as you even try to put your baby down for a sleep because he very quickly makes the association between pain and lying down in his cot. See Chapter 7 for more information on reflux.

Sleep basics

How much sleep?

How much sleep each individual baby needs can vary slightly, but the following table gives a general guide to an infant's sleep requirements. This table shows only the average number of hours a baby will need throughout each 24-hour period and is based on a full-term baby of average weight.

Baby's daily sleep requirements	
Age	**Average number of hours**
newborn	16–18
2 weeks	16–18
4 weeks	16–17
6 weeks	16–17
8 weeks	15.5–17
12 weeks	15–17
16 weeks	15–17
26 weeks (6 months)	15–16
1 year	14–15

The interesting point of this chart is that the typical sleep requirements of a baby from birth to one year show a very small and gradual reduction. In fact, many parents are amazed when they realize how much sleep a baby really does need.

Temperature

During the first few weeks your baby is unable to regulate his own body temperature and can easily overheat. It helps to manage this by keeping a check on the temperature in his room and using appropriate bedding.

Ideally, the temperature in your baby's room should be no higher than 21°C and no lower than 16°C, though in some houses it can be very difficult to maintain a steady temperature throughout both day and night.

Where possible I would advise you to try to keep your baby's room cooler rather than hotter by closing the curtains to block out direct sunshine, turning off radiators, opening windows where it is safe to do so and keeping the room well ventilated.

Bedding

To help regulate your baby's temperature, make sure that all bedding used in the cot is 100 per cent cotton. This also helps alleviate any possible problems with allergic reactions to man-made fibres or any skin sensitivity that your baby may have or develop. Studies have shown that the use of cot bumpers, cot duvets and pillows is not advisable. In the early weeks the good old-fashioned sheet and blanket are best for your baby. However, baby 'sleeping bags' or 'grow-bags' are becoming increasingly popular. These are advertised as being safe to use from birth and there seems to be little research to show otherwise; in fact, their use is now recommended and, as long as you choose a brand that is 100 per cent cotton and ensure you have the correct tog-rating for the changing seasons and also for your environment, they can be safely used. However, my advice is still to use a sheet and blanket in the very early weeks, as this helps your baby to feel more secure when he is tucked in snugly. Then from 6–8 weeks old change to using a sleeping bag.

Swaddling

You may choose to swaddle your baby by wrapping him in a soft, cotton sheet before putting him in his cot. Again, there is much varying advice about this method, so it really is up to individuals to form their own opinion. Personally, I do advise that swaddling a new baby can help him feel more secure and therefore able to settle better when it is time to sleep. There are many ready-made swaddles that you can buy; they come with instructions for use. Do make sure that the fabric used is 100 per cent cotton and avoid any man-made fibre. When you swaddle your baby, my advice is to put his arms crossed over his chest rather than straight down by his side as the latter is such an unnatural position and babies like the comfort of snuggling into the foetal position.

Swaddling your baby may also help to reduce the impact of the startle reflex. This is a natural reflex that occurs in young babies, causing them to make a sudden, jerky movement as if they have been startled by a loud noise. It can occur throughout sleep and babies can easily be woken or disturbed as their arms thrash around. Swaddling your baby with his arms across his chest lessens the impact, thus aiding undisturbed sleep. I would also suggest that you aim to stop swaddling your baby by 6–8 weeks, as the effect of the startle reflex should be much reduced by this age. By now he will probably be able to wriggle his arms free anyway and is likely to be more comfortable sleeping without the confines of the swaddle.

Nightclothes

The temperature in your baby's room and the bedding you have chosen to use will dictate what nightclothes he needs to wear – the table opposite provides a rough guide. Again, always opt for clothing that is 100 per cent cotton and use a couple of thin layers rather than one thick one, as this encourages a better circulation of air round the body. Research shows that a baby produces 40 per cent of his body heat in his head and will then lose 85 per cent of the generated heat through his head and face. This is the only way he can regulate his own temperature, therefore it is very important that his head remains uncovered during all sleep times.

Regulation of daytime temperature

An important point to mention here is that babies can overheat during the day as well as at night. Many parents ask me why their baby seems to hate his car seat. The main reason, I have discovered, is that many babies simply get too hot in their car seats and quickly build up an aversion. Even when it is cold outside, nowadays most cars are heated and get warm very quickly, so a baby dressed in a warm coat or covered with cosy blankets can easily overheat. On top of this, babies fit very snugly into their car seats which are often made of man-made materials and do not allow for much air circulation, all contributing to keeping the baby warm.

This also applies to shops. Outdoors your baby may be well wrapped up in the pram and then become too hot, as many shops today are well heated and completely under cover.

Temperature, bedding and nightclothes

Temperature	Tog-rating of bedding	Short-sleeved vest	Long-sleeved vest	Sleep suit without feet	Sleep suit with feet	Extra layer
very cold (below 16°)	2.5		✓		✓	✓
cold (around 16°)	2.0	✓			✓	
warm (17°–20°)	1.5	✓		✓		
hot (21°)	1.0		✓			
very hot (22° and above)	cotton sheet	✓				

Which room and which bed?

Where your baby should sleep is a much discussed, contentious issue and every healthcare professional has a different opinion. The most common are:

❍ In a separate cot or Moses basket in your room for at least six months.
❍ In a separate cot or Moses basket in your room for a few weeks.
❍ In a bedside crib with direct access to your bed for as long as needed.
❍ Sleeping in bed with you for as long as he wishes.
❍ In a separate cot or Moses basket, in his own room from the first week or two.

Whichever option you decide to use, you can be sure that someone will have, and give you, their opinion on it! Truly, though, the decision on where your baby should sleep is ultimately down to you. Therefore:

❍   Trust your own judgement.
❍   Look at your individual family requirements.
❍   Consider your residential situation.
❍   Follow your own instincts.
❍   Try to keep a rational perspective.
❍   Start as you mean to go on. For example, if you have your baby in bed with you for the first three months and then try to transfer him to his cot, he is likely to object. If you find yourself in this situation, see Chapter 6, which explains how to use my reassurance sleep-training technique.
❍   And do what you feel is right for you and your baby.

My suggestion is to put your baby in his own room within the first few weeks, or as soon as you feel comfortable doing so. I advise this for the simple reason that you and your baby will not be disturbing each other throughout the night and so will have a much more peaceful sleep. Babies rarely sleep without making some noise: they often whimper, snuffle, snort or even cry out, and many parents are continually woken by these sounds. As adults we also often snore, talk or mumble in our sleep and the rustle of the duvet or a creaky bed can sound quite loud in the silence of the night, risking disturbing the baby and causing him to wake. When he stirs within his sleep cycles, knowing that you are there and hearing your night-time noises may encourage him to wake rather than to settle himself back to sleep. Also, if you are breastfeeding he will probably be able to smell your milk and will be inclined to wake more frequently for a little snack even though he may not be properly hungry and ready for a full feed.

Alison says . . .

It is entirely up to you to decide where your baby should sleep. However, I must point out that when following my plan the best results are achieved when the baby sleeps in his own room.

The type of bed you choose for your baby is again a matter of individual preference. Many parents choose to use a Moses basket or crib for the first weeks and then transfer to a larger cot as he gets bigger. When you feel your baby is ready to make this transition, it is a good idea to put the Moses basket in the cot for a few nights so that he can gradually get used to his new surroundings. However, it is not necessary to use a Moses basket at all – you can put your baby straight into his cot from the start. Some parents use only a cot-bed, although these are quite large and possibly a newborn could feel somewhat 'exposed' by the space around him. You can overcome this and create a cosier environment by sectioning off and using only one end. Do be careful not to use anything soft, such as pillows or cushions, to divide the bed; use a specially designed cot-divider.

Bedtime for baby

It is important for parents who want to follow this plan to establish a happy bedtime routine to which both you and your baby will look forward at the end of each day. Not only does it set the pattern for a healthy association with nighttime sleeping, but it also means that you have the evenings free for some much needed 'adult-only' time. Much as you may adore your baby, his bedtime often comes with a certain amount of relief at the end of a busy day.

It can be a tempting prospect to cuddle up on the sofa in front of the TV with your baby snoozing in your arms throughout the evening, keeping him up with you until you go to bed. However, there will come a time when you would like your evenings to yourself, but your baby may now have other ideas and may protest loudly when you suddenly try to put him to bed in the early part of the evening. You may not realize that after, say, six weeks of staying up with you he will have already learned that this is normal procedure and may object to his habits being changed.

It may seem harsh to be putting your baby to bed on his own from the very early days, but within a short space of time he will come to accept the regular bedtime as part of his normal daily routine. This will have the added benefit that the set bedtime will continue through his toddler years and beyond.

Questions frequently asked about sleep

Q   *Why is it that I hear every noise our baby makes during the night but my husband never even hears the crying? In fact, if he offers to do the night feed there seems little point as I have to wake him up when I hear our baby cry for it.*

A   I think this scenario causes more disagreements between parents than any other. I have had countless mums ask me the same question and they are convinced that their partner is just being lazy and pretending not to hear the baby crying so that he doesn't have to get up! There are a few contributing factors that I have come up with through research, hands-on experience and conversations with many fathers.

The main reason is (and sorry for this, girls) that men are not physiologically programmed to react instinctively to a baby's cry as they do not produce the maternal hormones that link a mother to her baby. Some men who genuinely do not hear the crying when they are asleep believe it is because they know the mum is going to get up because she is breastfeeding, so they are not needed and can therefore switch off. But they do also say that if for some reason they are left in charge they do hear the baby and wake up as necessary. Others have been very honest and admitted that they do hear the crying sometimes but are able to ignore it and carry on sleeping in the knowledge that their partner will get up and see to the baby as needed. Some men, quite simply, are not hands-on dads, preferring to leave babycare to the mum as it is 'her job'. But then to be fair, there are also many men who are even more sensitive to the crying than the mother and want to respond to each and every whimper.

Q   *My husband does not get home from work until after 7.30 most evenings and will not see our baby all week if he goes to bed at 7pm. What can we do?*

A   Sadly, this is a common problem for a lot of busy families. In the early weeks, though, it is doubtful that your baby will be in bed at 7pm on the dot and he may still be finishing his feed or having that last cuddle before finally settling into his cot a little later into the evening.

It is very difficult for working parents who may see their baby for only a few minutes before bedtime as they arrive home from work, especially as this needs to be a quiet time. It may also be difficult not to overstimulate an already tired baby at this time of the evening. Some people, however, adapt the routine to fit in with their lifestyle and may adopt a slightly later bedtime by basing their day on the timing of 8am to 8pm instead of the suggested 7am to 7pm. However, it is strange that once this plan is established and the baby is sleeping through the night it doesn't seem to matter what time he wakes up in the morning – he will always be ready for his bed by 7 in the evening. Further to this, you have to take into account who actually benefits from keeping a baby up late to spend a few minutes with the returning parent, when all he really needs is to sleep. It is a harsh fact of a busy worklife that some parents get to spend quality time with their children only at weekends or on days off.

Q   *Our baby is six weeks old and we have been invited to dinner at a neighbour's house. We have already put a bedtime routine in place and our baby is usually in bed asleep by around 7.30pm. We don't want to mess up his routine, but we can't face leaving him with a babysitter. What would you suggest?*
A   This is a very good example of how this flexible routine can work and the benefits you can reap from establishing set sleep times for your baby at an early stage.

Carry out your usual bedtime routine. Put your baby into his nightclothes and give him his last feed, then settle him into the pram or carrycot. You can then take him with you for the evening, put him in a quiet room at your neighbour's and hopefully, because he is used to sleeping at this time, he will sleep quite happily. When you get home you can then transfer him to his cot for the rest of the night. If he does happen to wake, though, persevere and try to re-settle him, offering a feed only if really necessary.

Q   *We have been putting our baby to bed around 7pm since Week 1. He is now ten weeks old and still cries for around 10–15 minutes before going to sleep, but then he does sleep all through the night. Is this normal and is there anything we can do?*

A   Really there is no such thing as 'normal' – all babies are individuals and will display different behaviour patterns. Although he cries, your baby does eventually go to sleep and then sleeps through the night. This indicates that there is little wrong and I would suggest that it is just his way of winding down as he prepares to sleep. It is fairly common behaviour and nothing to worry about. I would advise little or no intervention to try to stop him crying as this may only disturb him, thus prolonging the time it takes him to go to sleep rather than comforting him.

Cot death and sleeping position

Research, advice and up-to-date statistics on cot death are readily available on the internet from the Foundation for the Study of Sudden Infant Death Syndrome. Many other reports and studies are also readily available to read. I believe it is up to each individual parent and carer to access the advice and information provided and to be aware, as I am, of the guidelines given.

> ### Alison says . . .
>
> I recently read a very interesting book called *The Cot Death Cover-up?* which disproves most of the common risk factors associated with cot death today.[6] It is well worth spending some time to read the author's proven theories.

Sadly, around 300 babies die suddenly and unexpectedly in the UK every year. Cot death can happen to any baby, but those aged between one and four months, premature babies, low-birth-weight babies, those suffering from gastro-oesophageal reflux or other underlying health issues, and male babies are most at risk.

Babies who die from cot death appear to die painlessly in their sleep. Many cases seem to occur during the night, but it can also happen during any other period of sleep, such as in the pram or even in a carer's arms.

Although the current recommended practice of laying babies on their backs to sleep has undoubtedly saved lives, there is growing concern among parents who are having to seek professional help to resolve sleeping problems in babies who simply cannot sleep comfortably on their backs. Most commonly, a baby suffering from gastro-oesophageal reflux will have difficulty sleeping on his back because when he lies down the weak sphincter muscle and valve in his stomach relax and allow the food and gastric acid to reflux into the oesophagus, thus causing severe pain as the acid burns the soft internal tissue. In my experience, these babies may benefit from a different sleep position. For further information and my views on some cot deaths possibly being linked to acid reflux, see Chapter 7.

Another major concern is the increasing number of babies who develop positional plagiocephaly, commonly known as 'Flathead Syndrome', as a result of constant pressure on the baby's soft skull from lying in the Back-to-Sleep position. It is said that this malformation will naturally correct itself as the baby grows, but increasingly this appears not to be the case: many toddlers and children continue to have a misshapen or flattened area on their heads which will last for the rest of their lives. In fact, to combat this growing problem, a number of clinics that specifically treat this condition have opened in the UK during the last few years. Treatment consists of the baby having to wear a corrective helmet for 23 hours every day for anything up to six months. Although the treatment is very successful, it is available only on a private basis and costs a substantial amount of money – but surely the fundamental question should be 'Why is it needed in the first place?' In my view this is a very real and serious problem that needs to be addressed. I believe the best way to avoid it happening is to settle a baby to sleep on alternate sides for the first few weeks or months, then as he grows and is able to roll over and move around to let him sleep in his preferred position, which will often be on his front.

If you do decide to try a different sleep position for your baby to avoid or combat the conditions mentioned above, then I would advise you to research the use of an under-mattress breathing sensor. This will monitor your baby's movements and sound an alarm if his breathing dips to an unacceptably low level or stops completely, thus alerting you in time to avoid a possible cot death. Be aware, however, that these monitors are effective only for babies up to twelve or eighteen months old, depending on the brand you buy. Also available on the market are completely portable 'breathing effort and movement' baby monitors which clip to the front of a baby's nappy and can be kept in place 24/7. Considering that cot death can occur at any time of day or night, wherever the baby is sleeping, these monitors could help to reduce the number of deaths still further. They work regardless of sleep position, have no dangerous electrical wires and the battery has a twelve-month lifespan. They have been tested in some neo-natal units with very positive results and I would urge the government to research their effectiveness with a view to issuing them for widespread use.

Alison says . . .

One baby lost to cot death is one too many, and if these monitors reduce the risk even further then their use has to be advocated.

Most parents today do seem to favour the use of a sound monitor, especially if the baby is sleeping in his own room. These are very useful, though not entirely necessary, as you may be surprised how easy it is to become attuned to your baby's noises without one. If you do decide to use a sound monitor, I advise you to have it on a low sound setting during the night, otherwise every little snuffle and snort your baby makes will be amplified to such a level that you will be disturbed all night long. Rest assured that even with the monitor set low you will be able to hear when your baby really needs your attention.

Mum's the Word . . .

Elsa sort of slept through the night from about eight weeks. However, she was on her back and thrashed about in her sleep and was very hard to settle, and she still always seemed so tired. She was diagnosed with reflux and we were then told to try propping her up during sleep, but this was really of no help. We then started a course of some reflux medication which helped ease her discomfort, but she was still so restless and uncomfortable during the night.

After consulting Alison we bought an under-mattress monitor and then put Elsa on her tummy to sleep. Bingo – what a difference! It was amazing to watch her in sleep – I could tell she was so much more comfortable and totally at rest.

We never looked back from that moment and it was tummy all the way.

S. S.

Structured daytime sleeps

On average, children will have a daytime sleep up to the age of three years, with some continuing until four and others giving it up as early as two years.

During the early weeks, when your baby is sleeping between each feed and seems unaware of his surroundings, there may seem little point in putting him back to bed during the day. However, to help establish a structured pattern of daytime sleeps it is best to put your baby back to bed for at least one or two naps when you are at home. If this is implemented during the first few weeks it will become an established part of his routine and will continue as an accepted practice for as long as he needs a daytime sleep. As a general rule, my advice is to put your baby down for a sleep in his bed after Feed 1 and again after Feed 2.

However, this does not mean that you must be tied to the house every day for these sleeps, as this routine is designed to be flexible. If the structured sleeps are established during the days when you are at home, your baby will have become so used to sleeping at these times that he should be able to sleep in other surroundings. For instance, when you are out for the day your baby can sleep in his pram, the car seat, maybe a sling or any other suitable place. If you are planning a journey, it is a good idea to try to arrange your travel to coincide with his naps. For example, after Feed 1, instead of putting him to bed, settle him into the car seat at his usual nap time and he can sleep while you are driving.

The following table gives an approximate daily feeding and sleeping routine for the first year. The daytime sleeps are often the last thing to fall into place when following this plan. It really is advisable to be as disciplined as possible in the early weeks and get the naps established within your feeding structure. As a general rule, most babies are ready to go down for their first nap of the day about 1½ hours after they have woken in the morning. In the early weeks you may be starting the day with your baby at any time between 6am and 8am, based on his demand for nighttime feeds, so the times that I have given in the table are only approximate and you will need to adapt naps to suit accordingly. You may have to fit in an extra nap or leave your baby asleep for longer in order to get back on track with your routine. For instance, if you had to start your day with Feed 1 at 6am, your baby is likely to need his first nap at 8am. If he then stays asleep until 10am you can wake him for Feed 2 and be back on schedule. If he wakes at 9am from his nap, however, you may have to feed him earlier than 10am and then hope to catch up later in the day, always aiming for bedtime at around 7pm.

Due to the daily variations that can occur, it is a good idea to keep a record of your baby's feeds and sleeps (see page 114). You will find some blank charts at the back of this book which you can fill in to begin your diary.

Alison says . . .

Always try to wake your baby during the day to stay on schedule for feed times.

Feed/sleep patterns, 1–12 months

	4 weeks	8 weeks	12 weeks	16 weeks	26 weeks	52 weeks
7am	feed	feed	feed	feed	feed	feed
8am				solids?*	solids	breakfast
8.30am	nap till 10am	nap till 10am	nap till 10am			
9am				nap till 10.30am	nap till 10am	
10am	feed	feed				
11am	nap till 1pm	nap till 1pm	feed	feed		
11.30am					small feed and/or solids	
12pm			nap till 2.30pm	nap till 2.30pm	nap till 2.30pm	lunch
12.30pm						nap till 2.30pm
1pm	feed	feed				
3pm	nap till 4pm	nap till 4pm	feed	feed	feed	
4pm	feed	feed				
4.30pm			nap till 5pm	nap till 5pm		
5pm	nap till 5.30pm	nap till 5.30pm		solids?*	solids	supper
5.30pm	top-up feed?	top-up feed?				
6.30pm	bath	bath	bath	bath	bath	bath
7pm	feed	feed	feed	feed	feed	feed

* I often advise introducing solids earlier than the recommended six months and suggest trying small amounts at 16–20 weeks onwards.

It may seem slightly restricting in the early weeks to put your baby back to bed for his first and second sleeps of the day, but if you can establish these sleeps at home you will reap the benefits in the months to come. As a new mother you can also use these nap times as an opportunity to get some much-needed rest yourself. It is also important for you to be out and about with your baby, meeting friends, shopping or going to groups, etc., and you should be able to adapt your baby's nap times to fit in with your outings.

Questions frequently asked about daytime naps

Q   *Do I always need to be at home for nap times during the day so that my baby can sleep in his cot?*
A   No, not necessarily. In the first few weeks when you are at home more often than not, do try to get the nap times established. You can then be more flexible about where your baby will sleep, and when out and about he should be able to sleep in his pram or car seat. Many families that have followed this plan have mentioned how well their babies have adapted when they have been on holiday, some even taking their midday nap in a sun-tent on the beach!

Q   *I have heard that I should not let my baby sleep for longer than 45 minutes in the morning or sleep at all after 4pm, but must keep him awake until bedtime. My baby seems to want to sleep more than this and it is very distressing trying to keep him awake. What should I do?*
A   LET HIM SLEEP! In my opinion a new baby can never have too much sleep and if kept awake will often become overtired and unhappy. Following my daytime feeding and sleeping pattern, you only need to wake your baby during the day to fit in with the 3-hour feeding schedule, otherwise leave him to sleep. Trying to keep your baby awake after 4pm will not ensure that he settles more easily at bedtime; in fact, it will often have the opposite effect and you may experience great difficulty when trying to settle him for the night. Also, it may make the whole bath, feed and bedtime routine distressing for you both, as your baby may well be extremely irritable and too tired to enjoy it.

Q *How long should I leave my baby after he has woken from a nap during the day to see if he will go back to sleep?*

A There are many points to take into consideration here and you need to learn to trust your judgement and make your own decisions accordingly. As all babies are individuals and each situation will be slightly different, there is no hard and fast rule that can be applied. It will depend on how long your baby has been asleep, what time of day it is and what sort of cry he is making. The following checklist should help you understand what your baby is saying and whether he is likely to settle himself back to sleep or needs some of your attention.

○ Has he got wind? Maybe he has just had a feed, fallen asleep straight away and woken up 15 minutes later. Try picking him up, wind him, then re-settle him again with the minimum of fuss.
○ Refer to the 'crying scale' on pages 174–5 and decide whether he needs attention or not based on his level of cry.
○ Maybe he has been asleep for over an hour and it is nearing the next feed time. In this situation it is unlikely that he will go back to sleep as he may be starting to feel hungry.

Q *My baby refuses to go down for his daytime sleeps and cries as soon as I try to lay him down. What can I do?*

A As a general rule, most babies should be able to feed well and therefore have little trouble when put down for a nap. If your baby is struggling to do this and seems very distressed, there is usually a reason and you will need to assess his behaviour to ascertain the root of the problem. Once you have checked that it is none of the obvious reasons – hunger, wind, dirty nappy, too hot or too cold – you might find it helpful to keep a log of his behaviour for a couple of days; this may then help you to understand where the problem is coming from. I would always advise you to have your baby checked by your GP and discuss the symptoms with him. In some cases I have found it to be a low-grade ear infection that is causing the problem; more often it can be attributed to a certain amount of digestive discomfort caused by a reflux issue from which your baby maybe suffering. See Chapter 7 for more information on this common complaint.

Sleep troubleshooting

The following common problems often crop up during the first year.

Frequent night-waking

If your baby is still waking frequently throughout the night and does not seem to be accepting the routine you are trying to establish, then it will be necessary to look back through your diary and try to find out why. Check that he is feeding well during the day, having plenty of wet and dirty nappies and gaining weight steadily. On average, a newborn baby should put on at least 120g (4oz) each week for the first couple of months. If your baby's weight gain is less than this on a regular basis, then he may be waking at night due to hunger. You will need to look at your chosen feeding method and increase the amount of milk he is taking by either giving him a longer time at the breast or introducing some top-up feeds from the bottle. If formula-feeding, increase the amount of feed offered. If your baby doesn't appear to feed well and you cannot get him to take more milk, it could be a reflux problem which means that, as well as being hungry at night, he may be suffering from acid heartburn which will cause him to wake (see Chapter 7 on reflux). I suggest you also read Chapter 6, which explains how to use my reassurance sleep-training technique, to discover more about sleep and how to avoid or overcome any problems.

Early-morning waking

This is a very common problem and can sometimes be quite difficult to resolve. However, if the early-morning waking occurs when your baby is around six weeks old and he has slept through the night from bedtime to the early hours – say, 5am – then see pages 103–8 on nighttime feeds, which explains how to reduce the need for this early-morning feed. As this process takes place, your baby should adapt fairly easily and be able to sleep through the early hours before waking for his first feed of the day. If you have successfully managed to remove all night feeds but your baby is still waking at around 5am, then you will need to try to ascertain the reason for this so you can address the problem accordingly.

○   Check that your baby is regularly getting enough daytime sleep. If not, see page 83 on structured daytime naps or Chapter 6 on sleep-training.

○   Some advisers are adamant that early-morning waking will be due to the fact that the room is not dark enough and that you should use a blackout blind to ensure total darkness. However, I believe your baby needs to learn to sleep in any environment and if he becomes used to total darkness he will be unable to sleep in rooms with ordinary curtains when you travel or stay with relatives.

○   Logically, you may think that if your baby is constantly waking in the early hours you need to put him to bed later in the evening. Surprisingly, this in fact has the opposite effect and will cause your baby to become overtired. Remember, lack of sleep causes overtiredness and disturbed nights, while more sleep leads to better-quality sleep and longer nights. The more sleep your baby has the better and for some cases of early-morning waking I would suggest putting your baby to bed earlier rather than later. It often solves the problem.

○   If your baby is waking early and just 'chatting' for 10 minutes or so but then happily going back to sleep, I would advise you to let well alone as your intervention may prompt him to think it is time to start the day.

○   During the first few weeks of implementing this plan the times that your baby may wake for the first feed of the day can be quite erratic and you may often be starting your day at around 6am. But usually by around three months, when your baby has been sleeping through the night for some time, his sleep patterns become really well established and any early-morning waking should naturally disappear as he sleeps 12–13 hours each night.

○   However, if your baby is waking in the early hours and crying to the point that you need to tend to him, then see Chapter 6 to resolve this problem.

Overtiredness

Few parents realize that overtiredness can have an extremely detrimental effect on their baby. Also, the signs and symptoms of a baby being overtired are often misread. An overtired baby may:

- become very irritable
- appear to become 'excited' and hyperactive
- thrash around with arms and legs flailing
- pull at his hair and scratch at his face
- cry or even scream inconsolably
- refuse to be comforted
- not readily accept a feed
- make himself sick through pent-up tension
- not be able to fall asleep easily

Mum's the Word . . .

My baby would cry so much in the evenings that I thought she just hated the fact that it was bedtime and I would hold her, try to feed her, sing to her and even put the TV on to try to calm her down. Absolutely nothing worked and one evening she was crying so much that I stripped her off as I was convinced something must be digging into her or her nappy was somehow pinching her!

I was utterly amazed, after speaking with Alison, to discover that she was just simply overtired. Alison advised me to just put her into the cot and leave her. I felt awful and was convinced she would not settle, but within 15 minutes she had stopped screaming, calmed down and was fast asleep! Bedtime is still sometimes a struggle, but by encouraging longer naps during the day we are resolving the problem and my baby goes to bed at 6.30pm most evenings without any fuss at all.

A. F.

If your baby has become overtired and displays any of the above symptoms, your natural reaction will be to try to comfort and console him, but often the best course of action is to put him to bed so that he can calm down and go to sleep. Often the more you try to pacify him the worse the situation can become. It may seem harsh just to put him into bed while he is so upset, but it is often the best thing to do and you may be surprised at how quickly he calms down, whereas if you keep trying to comfort him and stop him crying it just fuels his frustration.

If your baby has reached the point of being so overtired that he refuses his last feed at bedtime, then you may just have to put him to bed without it. Sometimes in this situation the more you try to get him to take the feed the more he will resist and it is better to resolve the issue by putting him to bed rather than to continue with the battle. After he has gone to sleep, should he happen to wake within the next hour you could then offer him a feed again, as he will be calmer having been asleep even if only for a short time. I would not recommend that you wake him for a feed during the night and if this means he doesn't feed until morning, try not to worry – he will come to no harm through missing one feed.

Obviously, there will not be a positive outcome should this situation occur on a regular basis, so if your baby is often reaching this level of over-tiredness then you will need to adjust your routine and encourage him to have more sleep during the day. See pages 17–20 on sleep deprivation and also Chapter 6.

Sleeping away from home

As I have already mentioned, if you encourage good sleep habits with your baby from a very early age, you will rarely experience any major problems and when you are on holiday or staying away from home your baby should still sleep well in the new environment. Where possible, aim to keep your usual bedtime routine in place, as this can help to reassure him that life is carrying on as normal even though you are away from home. It can help to take with you the sleeping bag that your baby is used to and any other familiar comfort blanket, muslin square or sheet that he may curl up with when going to bed at night.

If your baby sleeps in his own room at home you might feel worried about disturbing his sleep at night through having him in your room while staying in a hotel, for instance. There is little you can do in these circumstances except position the cot in a corner of the room as far away as possible from your bed. You may even be able to put the cot behind a screen, chest of drawers or wardrobe so that your baby cannot see you and will assume he is in his own room as usual.

If you travel to a country with a different time zone, you will need to adapt your routine and aim to get your baby on to local time as quickly as possible. The best way to achieve this is to use the same rule for your baby as you adopt for yourself: as soon as you get on to the plane, set your watch to the local time of the country you are visiting and carry on from that point with your baby's usual feeding and sleeping pattern. This may mean introducing an extra feed or sleep to stretch out the hours, but it usually falls into place fairly easily within a day or two.

In my experience, it is often quite easy to make the change on to the new time zone but harder to revert back to your usual schedule when you return home. Try to allow yourself a few free days when you arrive back so that you and your baby can re-adjust gradually. If you are going somewhere where the difference is only 1 or 2 hours, you may decide to leave your baby's routine set at the UK time, which can make life easier all round!

See Chapter 6, which explains how to use the reassurance sleep-training technique, as you may need to apply this when coping with different time zones if your baby's sleeping pattern becomes somewhat erratic.

Teething and sleep

To be honest, I rarely find that teething troubles will upset your baby's sleep pattern if you have been following this sleep plan from the early weeks. A baby who learns to sleep through the night from a young age is less likely to be disturbed in the later months when he starts teething as he will have become accustomed to sleeping so deeply that this slight discomfort should not bother him. The onset of teething is often quoted as the reason for a baby not sleeping through the night, but this can be a misrepresentation of the truth and should not be used as an excuse for why a baby is still waking at night. It is more likely that the baby has not been in a routine and has not learned to sleep well from Day 1.

If an older baby has woken in the night and you feel he is in real discomfort from teething, you may need to give him some Paracetamol-based pain relief, or use a teething gel or powders to alleviate the discomfort. It is better to stay in the baby's room with him until you can re-settle him rather than being tempted to take him to your bed for the rest of the night. Many parents have unwittingly initiated ongoing sleep problems in this kind of situation. You may need to offer your baby a drink of water after administering the medication, then as the pain subsides you should be able to re-settle him fairly easily.

Illness and sleep

If your baby is unwell he may not be able to sleep properly and you may need to give him attention throughout the night. As mentioned above, it is better to stay in the baby's room while he needs you rather than taking him into your bed. Even if he has been unwell throughout the day and hasn't taken much feed, it should not be necessary for you to re-introduce a feed during the night. Do offer a drink of water where appropriate, however, to keep him hydrated.

It is often after a bout of illness that sleep problems can occur, because your baby quickly gets used to your attention throughout the night and even when he is better he may continue to seek the comfort that you bring. If this does happen, see Chapter 6 to understand how to implement the reassurance sleep-training technique, which will help you and your baby get back on track as soon as possible once he has recovered.

If your baby has a cold and/or a cough, it may help to raise the head end of the cot slightly by placing some blocks under the feet. Saline nasal drops can be used to unblock stuffy noses and the use of a small vaporizer or humidifier can also help. There is little else that can be done to relieve the symptoms and you may experience a few disturbed nights until your baby recovers, but during this time make every effort to keep him in his own room, tend to his needs with the minimum of fuss and, as far as possible, stay within the boundaries of your routine.

During the night, if your baby develops a slight temperature and appears too hot, give him a dose of Paracetamol in accordance with the manufacturer's instructions and remove a layer or two of bedding or clothing to help bring his temperature down. Do remember that your own body heat will increase his temperature if you hold him closely for too long while trying to comfort him. It is best to try to lay him down, hold his hand or stroke his head to give him your reassurance while his temperature drops. A cool, damp cloth placed on his forehead for a few minutes or so can also help reduce a fever. If any symptoms persist or get worse, it is best to seek medical advice straight away.

☆ *Alison's Golden Rules* ☆

1 Never wake your baby at night unless you need to do so for medical reasons.

2 Establish a bath and bedtime routine as soon as possible during the first few days.

3 As soon as you feel comfortable to do so, and wherever possible, put your baby in his own room.

4 Always try to put your baby into his cot awake and leave him to settle himself to sleep.

5 Avoid using sleep aids such as lights, mobiles, etc.

6 Try not to let your baby fall asleep on his feed, but rouse him gently before putting him into his cot.

7 When he stirs during the night, try to sit back for a few minutes and see whether he is going to re-settle himself before you rush to tend him.

8 Ensure that your baby is getting enough good-quality sleep during the day.

9 Persevere during the weeks that your baby is up twice between midnight and 5am for feeds. It does soon pass and you will be well on your way to the full 12 hours before long.

10 Try to resist the temptation to take baby into bed with you either to feed or comfort him, as it may soon become a habit that you will later find hard to break.

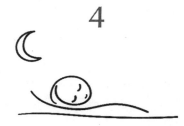

4

How to Implement the Sensational Baby Sleep Plan

Now that you have read the first three chapters, I hope that they will have given you enough knowledge and guidance on the basic feeding and sleeping issues that commonly crop up for new parents and that you will have decided that following this plan is the way forward for you and your baby. This chapter explains in detail the actual feeding schedule that you will be aiming to put in place on a daily basis; what you can expect in terms of night feeding with your newborn baby; and how the necessity for nighttime feeds gradually diminishes and then disappears by around Week 8. By this point, through following the advice as set out in my plan, you can expect your baby to be sleeping well for scheduled daytime naps, to be feeding efficiently during the day, to have an established bath and bedtime routine and to be sleeping through the night. When I talk of sleeping through the night I *always* mean the full 11–12 hours from 7pm to 6am or 7am – not 11pm to 6am or 7am as is often mentioned in other babycare books and methods.

Daytime feeds

In the early weeks most of your baby's waking hours will be spent feeding, so in order to avoid excessive night feeding it is important to structure and establish a good daytime feeding pattern. This routine works for a number of reasons, the main ones being that it helps establish a good feeding structure, helps to get your baby to sleep through the night from an early age and keeps him happy and content as he is never left to cry for food.

The plan follows a 3-hour feeding pattern during the day, which is based on the fact that after a full feed it will take approximately 2 hours for a newborn baby's stomach to digest and empty its contents. It is upon this physiological fact that I have based my plan and I rarely advise stretching a newborn baby's feeds to 4-hourly in the early weeks. Added to this, in the first month of life a baby will often be able to stay awake only for 1 hour at a time and will then need to sleep for about 2, hence feeding every 3 hours during the day provides the ideal feed:sleep ratio.

> **Mum's the Word . . .**
>
> ❜ Logan adapted to Alison's routine really well. He loved the structure and the 3-hour intervals ensured he was never crying through hunger, but always ready for each feed. ❛
>
> K. B.

It is helpful to think of each 24-hour period as two separate halves:

○   12 hours of day
○   12 hours of night

In my plan I use the timing:

○   7am–7pm = day
○   7pm–7am = night

During your 12 hours of day you will be aiming to fit in five feeds. Basing these on the 3-hourly schedule, they will be roughly timed at:

○   7am
○   10am
○   1pm
○   4pm
○   7pm

Please remember this is not so much about the actual time of the feeds, but more about the sequence of feeds and sleeps throughout the day. I do not want you to feel that you have to watch the clock rather than your baby! This is a flexible routine and you may have to adjust feed times to fit in with all the unexpected events of each new day. The table below shows how the feeding structure works and the following two examples suggest how to adapt your feeds when necessary:

A flexible structure for daytime feeds

Feed	Target time	Flexi-time	Note
Feed 1	7am	**6–8am**	Try to start the day no earlier than 6am and no later than 8am.
Feed 2	10am	**9–11am**	If baby has fed at, say, 6.15am and is then asleep at 9.15am (3 hours later), let him sleep till 10am to get back on target for the day.
Feed 3	1pm	**12 noon–2pm**	If this feed happens to be early, you can always fit in a quick top-up later on in the afternoon.
Feed 4	4pm	**3–5pm**	5–6pm is often 'unhappy hour'. Giving a small top-up at 5 or 5.30pm may help.
Feed 5	7pm	**6–8pm**	Always try to adjust feed times throughout the day so that you end up doing the bedtime routine and feed around 7pm.

Baby wakes at 5am and needs a feed Treat feeds before 6am as night feeds and put your baby back to bed directly afterwards. He may then not be ready to feed at 7am and you may both enjoy an extra hour of sleep, but do wake him around 8–8.30am and give another feed. If he is not that interested in this feed, don't push it but offer a feed again around 10–10.30am. You are then nearly back on track for the rest of the day. If he takes a good feed at 8.30am he may push through till 12 or even 12.30pm before needing the next feed and you can then try to push the next feed on to 3.30pm, give a small top-up feed at 5.30pm and then his usual bedtime feed at 7pm.

You have an appointment at 10am and the journey each way is 30 minutes Quite simply, I would advise you to wake your baby at 6am to start the first feed of the day, then feed at 9am before you leave for your appointment. Suppose you then get home at 11.30am and your baby is asleep, I suggest you leave him till as near 1pm as possible before feeding to get back on track. However, if he is unsettled on your return home and looking for a feed, do just feed him. He may then settle and sleep for quite a while and you can offer further feeds at 2–2.30pm with a top-up at 5pm and normal bedtime feed at 7pm.

As you can see, the feed times are always flexible. Every new day that you face with your baby will pose a slightly different scenario and mean that you need to make decisions on how to adapt his feed and sleep times according to that day's events, following your baby's signals of either hunger, tiredness or just being unsettled. As the days pass, your confidence will start to grow as you begin to make instinctive decisions based on your growing understanding of your baby's signals and what works best for you and for him.

You will find blank charts at the back of this book that you can use to start keeping a daily diary to chart your baby's progress.

> ### *Alison says . . .*
> Sometimes things will go smoothly and the day will pass with ease – but sometimes everything may seem to go pear-shaped. But don't panic! Tomorrow is another day and you can just add each experience to the ever-growing pile of parenting lessons.

To ensure that you can fit in the five daytime feeds, it will sometimes be necessary to wake your baby during the day. (See pages 83–7 for advice on structured daytime sleeps.) It can be tempting to leave him to sleep and let him wake of his own accord, but if he sleeps too long and doesn't eat enough during the day he will want to make up for it somewhere – and that will be during the night! I do appreciate that it can be very time-consuming to stick to 3-hourly feeds in these early weeks, but if you do persevere you will quickly reap the benefits as he sleeps all night by eight or ten weeks. You can then move on and drop to 4-hourly feeds during the day.

In the first few weeks a feed can easily take up to an hour and sometimes slightly more. By the time you have stopped to wind your baby a few times, had to change a nappy or two, spent time trying to get the latch right if you are breastfeeding, or just had to wait for your baby to show enough interest to start feeding, time can easily run away with you. I do advise, where possible, that you try to limit the actual feed time to around 60 minutes, otherwise each one can seem to run into the next. If it's your first baby, then you may enjoy the luxury of having plenty of time to focus on each feed. It's a different story, however, for subsequent babies with lively siblings running around and needing your attention.

Questions frequently asked about keeping feeding on track

Q   *What do I do if I cannot wake my baby fully and he seems too sleepy to take a daytime feed?*
A   There are many little things you can try, such as undressing him, changing his nappy, tickling his feet, changing the environment by moving from one room to another. However, sometimes he will just not be ready to wake up and there is nothing you can do except wait! Don't panic: feed him as soon as he is ready and adjust further feeding times accordingly. It may often seem that your baby is not following the feed times at all, but within a few weeks you and he will have established the pattern and it will all gradually fall into place.

Q   *I was late home and didn't start Feed 4 till 5pm. What shall I do?*
A   If your baby had a really good feed at 5pm, I would delay bathtime until around 7–7.30pm and start the bedtime feed after that. If he had only a small feed at 5pm, then keep to your normal bath and bedtime. However, amazingly enough, no matter what schedule is being followed on any particular day – for example one that is dictated by what time the baby wakes up – I often find that a baby is ready for his usual bedtime and will still want his feed even if he had Feed 4 later than usual.

Q   *I often find that my baby is unable to wait for his next feed. What shall I do?*

A   If you are breastfeeding this can be quite common in the first couple of weeks and if you need to offer an extra top-up feed or so during the day do just 'go with the flow' as this phase should soon pass. However, if your baby seems unable to take enough milk at each feed and is therefore consistently unable to fall into the 3-hour feeding plan, then there may be another reason and I would advise you to read pages 54–9 on troubleshooting feed problems and Chapter 7 on reflux. Always remember, though, that my plan is flexible, so if your baby is evidently hungry half an hour or so before feed time, then it's best to feed him and perhaps give a small top-up later on to get back on track for bedtime.

Nighttime feeds

When I talk about nighttime feeds I am referring to any feeds given after the bedtime feed at 7pm and before the first feed of the day at around 7am. Many newborn babies who are put straight on to this 3-hour feeding plan during the day very quickly settle into feeding 4-hourly at night during the first couple of weeks. However, some babies, especially those with a low birth weight or who have been born prematurely, will feed 3-hourly round the clock for the first week or two. Always wait for your baby to wake naturally before deciding whether he needs a feed or is just stirring within his sleep cycle. It is important not to respond too quickly to each noise he makes – as explained earlier, he may often cry out yet still be asleep, or even cry for a few minutes before settling himself back to sleep without your intervention. Your baby will quickly learn that he gets rewarded with attention as soon as he cries and if you react immediately to every whimper he will more easily be encouraged into frequent night-waking.

As the days go by, your baby should start to wake later each night for his first nighttime feed. It may then mean that for a week or two you are giving two feeds in the early hours – for instance, 12.30am and 4am. It may well be very tiring having to get up twice during the night, but it will be for only a short time. Very soon your baby will be sleeping for longer, with only one night feed at around 3am. To avoid two night feeds, many parents follow other advice and wake their baby at 11pm, thinking they will then get a less disturbed night – but it seldom happens this way. Instead your baby will quickly fall into the habit of waking himself for the feed at 11pm and may continue to do so for a number of months to come. Also, by waking your baby you are giving him food that his body does not require and stimulating his digestive system when it needs to be at rest.

When giving night feeds try to resist the temptation to take your baby into bed with you to feed him. It is far better to sit in a chair and carry out the feed with the minimum of fuss, keeping the lights low and nappy-changing only if necessary. Put him back to bed straight after the feed. If you are breastfeeding you will have more success using my plan if you follow this advice rather than feeding your baby while lying in bed. I also advise that very early on you begin to offer at least one of the night feeds from a bottle. In order to ensure that your milk supply gets established, it is best to feed from the breast at night for the first couple of weeks, but by Week 2 or 3 you can replace one of the night feeds with a bottle of expressed milk or formula. My reasons for this are:

○ It is often quicker to give a feed from a bottle, therefore reducing the amount of time you have to be up at night.
○ Somebody else can give the feed, allowing the breastfeeding mother to get more rest.
○ If you are breastfeeding but would like the alternative of using a bottle at any future stage, then you really *must* introduce your baby to the bottle in the first couple of weeks. Otherwise, later on, he may simply refuse to accept the bottle in favour of the breast and there will seem to be little option other than to continue with exclusive breastfeeding. See pages 49–54 for more information on weaning from the breast.
○ If you are still feeding from the breast at night your baby may continue to wake more frequently, knowing that he gets lovely cuddles snuggled up close to Mum during the feed. A bottlefeed, however, is not such an attractive prospect because he has little chance to prolong it by suckling for extra comfort.
○ As the need for nighttime feeds decreases, the contents of the bottle

can be gradually diluted to reduce your baby's reliance on nourishment during the night, thus helping him to sleep through. If you are feeding with expressed breast milk, it can be diluted by adding cooled boiled water, and if using formula you can begin to reduce the number of scoops you add to the usual amount of water. The dilution should be done over a couple of weeks, gradually increasing the ratio of water to milk and ending with just offering plain water if your baby is still waking. During this time also reduce the volume of diluted feed that you offer so that when it becomes a drink of plain water it will be only 30–60ml (1 or 2 fl. oz). See the tables on page 112, which explain the process in more depth. Do remember that it is safe to reduce the number of formula scoops you add to the water but never to increase them.

When your baby is sleeping through the night without requiring a night feed, you can choose one of the daytime feeds to replace with the bottle, thus keeping at least one bottlefeed in place during each day to ensure your baby's prolonged acceptance. It is entirely up to you which feed you choose. It may be dictated, for instance, by returning to work. Your baby may be having bottlefeeds while you are away during the day and you may feed from the breast first thing in the morning and then at bedtime. Usually, though, I advise using the bottle for the bedtime feed at 7pm. I have found this to work fairly well for a number of reasons:

○ It can provide a busy, working dad with the opportunity to have some contact and be involved with baby before bedtime.
○ After a long, tiring day, your breast-milk supply may be diminishing and may not be enough to sustain your baby throughout the night. You may decide still to offer the breast, but then to top up with a bottle of expressed milk or formula.
○ Babies are also very often tired after a long day and may not have enough energy to take a full feed from the breast. Most babies usually find it less tiring to take milk from a bottle.
○ It is usually quicker to give a bottlefeed, therefore giving you more free time each evening.
○ It gives you the opportunity to see how much milk your baby has

had and therefore to be confident that he should not require another feed till morning.

Mum's the Word . . .

❝ The sleep-training and routine go hand in hand to create a happy child. It gives them security and makes them less tired, which makes them less cranky, which means their behaviour is much better, so there is a lot of positive attention on which they thrive that subsequently encourages more positive behaviour. It's a virtuous circle! ❞

Y-L. L.

The table below shows how your baby's night feeds may progress during the first eight weeks. It is impossible to predict how each individual baby will behave throughout the night, so there will always be some variation in waking and feeding times.

Reducing night feeds		
Week	**Approximate time of feeds**	**Note**
Week 1	first feed between 10pm and midnight second feed between 1 and 3am	In this first week baby may wake more frequently and need three night feeds.
Week 2	first feed between 11pm and 1am second feed between 2 and 4am	If baby is already beginning to sleep for longer, make the most of it!

Week 3	first feed between midnight and 2am second feed between 3 and 5am	If baby is not yet stretching to these times, don't panic. He will get there eventually.
Week 4	first feed between 1 and 3am second feed between 4 and 5.30am	5am is the 'witching hour'. When baby wakes around this time you will need to adapt accordingly, by either giving a smaller or watered-down feed now, aiming to stay on track for Feed 1, or delaying feeding for as long as possible and starting your day by giving Feed 1 around 6am.
Week 5	one feed between 2 and 4am	Hopefully baby is now waking for just one nighttime feed.
Week 6	one feed between 3 and 4am	If at this point baby is still waking twice a night, then you have to make a stand, ignore his first waking and not feed him. There may be a few tears, but it won't last for long!
Week 7	one feed between 4 and 5am	Baby may now start to alternate between sleeping through and having one night feed.
Week 8	possibly no feeds at all	If baby is sleeping through, enjoy! If he is still insisting on one feed, then start to water it down by either putting in fewer scoops of formula or adding water to expressed breast milk. See tables, page 112, for more information on this.

Some babies adapt to this guide with ease; others need a little more encouragement. I do not suggest that you leave your baby crying for long periods at night, but it is important to leave him for a few minutes when he wakes to see whether he is going to settle himself back to sleep or not. Each night try to set a target time in your mind that you aim to reach before feeding your baby. For instance, if he has been waking for his first feed anywhere between 11 and 11.30pm for the last three nights, then set your target time as maybe 11.45pm or midnight and keep trying to lengthen the time before you give him a feed. As long as daytime feeds are on schedule and generally going well, a baby will not usually start demanding his feed the minute he wakes, but may moan and cry a little while dozing in between times before he really builds up to a full-blown hunger cry and demands his feed. Parents obviously have a natural instinct to pick up their baby as soon as he stirs, but I always advise leaving the baby for at least a few minutes before rushing to feed him, as more often than not he will settle himself back to sleep for a while.

Many parents find that their second and subsequent babies never learn to sleep through the night, because to try to prevent their toddler from being woken by the new baby's cries they quickly tend to each murmur and readily feed the baby to keep him quiet. This results in the baby learning that he receives attention and food as soon as he stirs, enjoying his own one-to-one time with Mum or Dad during the night and therefore having little incentive to sleep through. Although it is natural to feel anxious about your baby's cries disturbing your toddler, in my experience this is rarely the case: most older children will continue to sleep soundly. Also, if your partner has to get up early for work in the morning and needs to be able to sleep, I suggest the use of earplugs if necessary! Do remember that by following this plan your baby will be sleeping through the night within a matter of weeks and peace will (hopefully) be restored.

Mum's the Word . . .

When my third baby was born I was sure I knew what I was doing, but by Week 6 my baby was still waking three or four times each night wanting to feed. I couldn't work out why, so I called Alison for help and after some discussion she pointed out that maybe this new baby had already learned that the only one-to-one time she had with me was during the night. Having a very hectic daily life with my three- and one-year-olds to look after, I realized that apart from the necessary feeds, etc., my little baby hardly had any of my attention during the day at all – no wonder she was staying awake much of the night! After implementing Alison's plan and getting a bit of extra help from my family, I was able to re-train my baby to eat during the day, sleep during the night and we could spend more time together during the day. Alison is spot on when she says that babies are cleverer than we realize and are very aware of what is happening, even from day one!

H. C.

Questions frequently asked about night feeds and waking

Q *What happens if my baby needs a feed at night but doesn't wake for it?*
A   Unless you have been medically advised to feed your baby throughout the night, you *do not* need to wake him for a feed. In the early weeks he will wake of his own accord and you can give feeds as necessary. As a rough guide, your baby will need to be around 3.9kg (8lb 10oz) in weight before he has enough body mass to sustain sleeping through. This, though, doesn't mean that babies born at this weight or higher *will* sleep through from birth; you will still need to follow the night-feeding pattern set out in this plan.

Over the years some people have queried the practice of 'allowing' an eight-week-old baby to sleep 12 hours through the night without a feed – even suggesting it is unkind. But when using my daytime plan a baby should receive enough nourishment to sustain him throughout the night and if he does need a feed then he will wake for it. There is no part of this plan that suggests you do not feed a newborn baby at night when he really needs it. On the other hand, in my opinion it is totally unnecessary to wake a baby at night for a feed that he doesn't require, thus disturbing the development of his sleeping pattern.

Q *When my baby has woken up during the night, how long should I wait before going to feed him?*
A As I have said, I do not suggest leaving your baby to cry for long periods. However, I find it helps to imagine a 'crying scale', with 1 being the merest whimper and 10 being a full-on scream. When your baby reaches around 6 or 7 on the scale, that is the time he will probably need attention. (For more on my crying scale, see pages 87 and 174–5.) Amazingly, though, a baby may reach this level of cry but, by the time you have got up, used the bathroom or gone downstairs to get a bottle, he may already have gone back to sleep. There is no set timescale of how long you should wait before tending to your baby when he has woken, but by listening to him and using the crying scale you will soon learn to trust your own parental instincts and be able to make your own judgements with confidence.

Q *My baby is eight weeks old and is still waking at around 3am and expecting a feed. What shall I do?*
A Some babies may need a little more training to do without the last night feed completely. As long as your baby is feeding well during the day and is steadily gaining weight, you can start to dilute and reduce the volume of this night feed, making a gradual transition to eradicating it by following the guidelines in the table on page 112.

Q *My baby is now four months old and from nine weeks old he has been sleeping through the night without waking or feeding. Suddenly he has started to wake at night at around 2am and is sucking on his hand as if hungry. Should I offer him a feed?*

A   Babies can be unpredictable and, despite having been settled in a routine for several weeks, their habits can for some reason suddenly change. We may never discover what causes these changes, but in this case it could be due to the fact that your baby is hungry and not being sustained through milk alone. I would *not* advise you to re-introduce milk feeds at night but to look at his daytime feeding pattern with a view to increasing the amount of milk he takes, perhaps changing him on to a hungrier-baby formula or even starting to introduce some simple solid food such as baby rice. To understand how to re-settle your baby at night without giving a night feed, see Chapter 6 on the reassurance sleep-training technique.

Mum's the Word . . .

My baby had been waking up for a feed at 5am for ages when Alison explained how to water down the feed. I was absolutely amazed at how quickly this worked. Within five nights my baby was sleeping through and not waking for the feed at all.

K. W.

Diluting and reducing night feeds

Note This is a rough guide, which is easy to adapt as necessary and is based on a baby who is taking a 180ml (6 fl. oz) feed and starting at Week 8.

NB 30ml is equivalent to 1 fluid ounce

Nights	Breast milk:water		Water:formula scoops	
1, 2, 3	120ml	40ml	180ml	4 scoops
4, 5, 6	90ml	40ml	150ml	3 scoops
7, 8, 9	60ml	60ml	120ml	2 scoops
10, 11, 12	30ml	60ml	90ml	1 scoops
13, 14	Just a drink of water, no more than 60ml			

If you are exclusively breastfeeding and have chosen not to introduce a bottle at any stage, you could start to reduce the baby's time at the breast to try to encourage him to cease night-feeding. Again, this should be a gradual process. Use the chart below as a rough guide.

Nights	Length of feed	Reduction	New feed
1, 2, 3	45 mins	5 mins	40 mins
4, 5, 6	40 mins	5 mins	35 mins
7, 8, 9	35 mins	10 mins	25 mins
10, 11, 12	25 mins	10 mins	15 mins
13, 14	Try just offering a drink of water		

Your diary

Many mothers find it useful to note down feed and sleep times during each day, adding any comments as necessary. This can be beneficial for a number of reasons:

○ You may often find it hard to remember what happened at the last feed, let alone yesterday.

○ If you need to seek medical help or wish to discuss your baby's feeding pattern with anyone, then it can be very useful to be able to refer to a simple record.

○ When another baby comes along, some mothers find it useful to compare the notes they made for their first.

○ It can give you the encouragement to persevere with the plan, as it helps to show the progress of your baby's developing sleep pattern as the weeks pass.

Below is an example of a simple chart that you can devise to record your baby's progress and at the back of this book are some blank charts that you can fill in to begin your diary.

B = breast
L = left
R = right
EBM = expressed breast milk
F = formula
W = wet nappy
D = dirty nappy

Diary entry for a four-week old, mostly breastfed baby

Date/ time	Feed		Amount/ duration	Nappy	Comment
01/03/07					
7am	B	L	40 mins		
		R	10 mins	W/D	Fed well, slept for 1½ hours after feed.
10am	B	R	30 mins		
		L	15 mins	W	Bit fussy at feed, seemed agitated. Didn't settle easily for nap. Only slept 1 hour.
12.40pm	B	L	40 mins		
		R	20 mins	W/D	Much better feed, crashed out after and slept for 2 hours!
4pm	EBM		120ml/4oz	W/D	Fed well.
6.45pm	B	R	30 mins		
		L	20 mins	W/D	Fed OK. Very sleepy. Settled to bed OK.
2am	F		130ml	W	Slept well, settled back to sleep easily.
6.30am	B	R	40 mins		Woke at 5am! But dozed off again after 15 mins.
		L	10 mins	W/D	

Moving on to 4-hourly feeds

After around eight weeks your baby should have responded well to the plan, be sleeping through the night and no longer needing a night feed. Once he has consistently slept through for around 12 hours each night for at least two weeks, you can gradually start to reduce the number of daytime feeds by increasing the time between each feed from 3 hours to 4 hours. Your baby may very well indicate that he is ready for this change by losing interest in his 3-hourly feeds, not taking as much milk each time and generally appearing to be 'bored' by the whole feeding process. This may also cause him to stir during the night because he is actually hungry, having taken less milk during the day. If he is starting to wake at night again after sleeping through for a few weeks, look at his daily feeding schedule and adjust it accordingly rather than taking the backward step of re-introducing a nighttime feed.

There is no hard and fast rule about when your baby may be ready to drop a feed. Trust your own judgement and watch for signals from your baby that indicate he may be ready for this step. The following points are a guide to help you implement the change:

○ Decide on a day to begin and after the first feed try to distract your baby, perhaps by going for a walk. Aim to give him the next feed 30–60 minutes later than usual.

○ If you find that even after a few days your baby is distressed or unhappy while waiting for his feed, then go back to your original 3-hour plan and try again in a couple of weeks' time.

○ Moving on throughout the day, if your baby fed at 11am then went down for his daytime nap, aim to give his next feed at 3pm. Many babies cannot manage to last out until 3pm during the first few days of implementing the change, so you may need to feed him at 2.30pm instead.

○ Your baby may then struggle to wait until 7pm for his last feed of the day. You can either introduce a small top-up feed at 5pm (which, in effect, will shortly become 'teatime'), or start your bathtime routine a bit earlier so that you can feed him at 6.15 or 6.30pm with a slightly earlier bedtime to follow.

○ Often by this stage of moving to 4-hourly feeds, babies are ready for sleep and need to be in bed by 7pm. This makes it easier to move off the 3-hourly schedule and on to four feeds during the day, as the times of feeds naturally become 7am, 11am, 2.30pm and 6.30pm.

○ If you find that your baby is not able to enjoy his bathtime and cannot wait for his last feed, then you may decide to introduce the 'teatime top-up' at around 5pm. As the name implies, this will not be a full feed but perhaps just a few minutes at the breast or 90–150ml (3–5 fl. oz) of milk from a bottle. This should make the last part of your day together a happier time as your baby will not be irritable through hunger.

○ If your baby is nearing the age for weaning, you could introduce a solid food such as baby rice mixed with some of his usual milk as the teatime top-up and this will eventually become an established mealtime.

☆ *Alison's Golden Rules* ☆

1   Never wake your baby at night unless for medical reasons.

2   Always wake your baby during the day to stay on track with feeds.

3   Use my plan from day one, or as early as possible.

4   Don't get obsessed with the time on the clock. It is the regular sequence of feeds and sleeps that is important, not the actual down-to-the-minute timing of them.

5   Always introduce an end-of-the-day bath and bedtime routine as soon as it is possible to do so.

6   Where possible, do not immediately rush to feed your baby at his first whimper when he stirs at night.

7   Keep night feeds as calm as possible without too much interaction and settle your baby back to *his* bed as soon after the feed as you can.

8   Never wake your baby during the late evening to give the so called dream feed.

9   Persevere with daytime feeds to ensure your baby has taken enough milk at each feed to help sustain him longer at night.

10   Now reap the benefits of having used the Sensational Baby Sleep Plan and luxuriate in all the sleep-filled nights to come while still enjoying life with your happy and well-rested baby.

5

What to Expect: a Week-by-Week Guide

Much as I would like to give you a 'set script' to follow with your new baby, it is impossible to do so because like us, babies can be totally unpredictable at times and rarely do exactly the same thing from one day to the next. However, although allowing for the flexibility of daily life and taking into account each baby's individuality, my plan is relatively straight-forward to follow and most babies will adapt to it with ease. This chapter explains what you can expect from week to week with regard to the sleeping and feeding pattern outlined in this book.

> ### *Alison says . . .*
>
> I always expect the unexpected when dealing with each new baby.

Alongside some general information and explanations of the typical responses displayed by many babies following my plan, I have included a detailed case study – 'Cameron's Story' – to give a personal slant. It describes my family's experiences of using the plan when my grandson was born in January 2009. The charts recording his feeds and sleeps begin at Week 2, as during the first week it was almost impossible to chart anything because Cameron hardly fed or slept at all! The charts contain actual excerpts from the diary that his mother, Chelsea, kept and I have picked two days out of each week to use as typical examples of the events during that particular week.

Week 1

These first few days can pass by in a complete haze and I often think that new parents look somewhat like the proverbial startled rabbits in the headlights. I have lost track of the number of times that parents have exclaimed, 'OK, here we are at home with our new baby – but *what do we do now?*' Well, the answer lies right here, and the sooner you start to implement my plan the more easily you and your baby will settle down happily together.

Mum's the Word . . .

As a first-time mum I had no experience of establishing a baby routine and felt overwhelmed by all the contradictory advice in the numerous books I had read. Through two short phone conversations with Alison she not only diagnosed a mild reflux problem that I was unaware of as being responsible for his sleep-time restlessness, but also gave me some sensible advice on my routine that absolutely coincided with what my baby seemed to want to do. You don't feel like you are imposing a routine on your baby, rather encouraging him to do what he naturally wants to do (i.e. sleep!) within a daytime routine that gives you structure and confidence.

Practical, sensible advice that is not only in tune with your baby's natural patterns but also gives you your life back because they are happy little people by day and at night they SLEEP!

C. M.

As soon as you are able, whether you are still in hospital or at home, try to put your 3-hourly feeds in place during the day. Even before your milk has come in it is advisable to put your baby to the breast so that he can take the colostrum that is produced immediately after birth. Stimulating your breasts in this way will help to induce your milk supply. If you are bottlefeeding he should be able to take anywhere between 20ml and 90ml (0.7–3 fl. oz) per feed. Your baby needs to take frequent fluids, albeit in small amounts, to help flush through the meconium that is in his bowels after birth. After the meconium is passed, your baby's poos will gradually change to bright yellow, yellowy-green or yellowy-brown, depending on whether he has breast milk or formula or both. If he shows little interest in feeds, or if you are experiencing any problems in trying to feed him, then do make sure to ask your midwife, who should be on hand to help, and seek a further opinion if you are still worried in any way.

Did you know?

Meconium is a greenish-black, sticky, tar-like substance that builds up in the baby's bowel while he is in the womb and is then passed as 'first stools' in the first day or two after birth.

In these early days some babies are very sleepy and quite slow to feed, while others will actively look for food and want to feed as often as every 2 hours. Although I have advised you to implement a 3-hour feeding plan, I do know that this can be quite difficult for one reason or another during this first week and you may just have to 'go with the flow' until things begin to settle down as you head towards Week 2.

Do remember, as I have explained in Chapter 3, that babies are basically nocturnal when they are born and are likely to be more active during the night and sleepier during the day. That is why, as soon as possible after they are born, it is important to start waking them during the day for their feeds, but not during the night. Also, when you get home and have settled in, it is a good idea to put your bath and bedtime routine in place within this first week. This does not need to be complicated to begin with – a very quick wash and change of clothes before the last feed of the day will suffice.

Some babies may seem to be quite traumatized by birth and will need a lot of comforting before they are able to relax and settle into their new surroundings.

By the end of this first week you should find that your baby has started feeding and sleeping at regular intervals as you implement the plan. However, this may not be the case for some babies, as highlighted by our experiences with my grandson.

Cameron's Story

Three days after her eighteenth birthday my daughter, Chelsea, gave birth to a gorgeous baby boy – Cameron Jack. She is a single mum and still lives under my roof, so I have been closely involved with Cameron from the start, when I was present at his birth. Cam was born three weeks early, after an induced labour, weighing 3kg

(6lb 13oz) and was put to the breast straight away. However, he showed no interest at all and did not display the 'rooting reflex' at all during the next few days. Midwives said he was 'just sleepy', or that it was 'because of the pain relief used in labour', or that he was 'a boy and therefore a bit lazy', but things did not improve. One midwife expressed her concern at his lack of interest in feeding and advised that discharge from hospital should not go ahead until Cam had taken a substantial feed. However, after a change in the nurses' shift, Chelsea and Cam were discharged home 24 hours after birth.

The next three days were a mix of Cam screaming, Chelsea crying, Cam refusing to feed and rarely sleeping, and me looking after them both. As the days passed and Cam refused to breastfeed I tried to get him to take a bottle, but all he would do was suck three times, swallow, gag and choke, then scream. It took until Day 5 for a midwife to agree to come to watch him try to feed, after which she sent us straight to see the GP. We showed him a video of what happened when Cam tried to feed and he sent us to the paediatric unit at our local hospital.

Alison says . . .

Having experienced similar scenarios with many clients I thought I would be well prepared – but when it is your own, so to speak, nothing can prepare you for the emotional trauma you may encounter when dealing with a baby who won't feed.

During those first few days it was impossible to stick to any feeding plan and the only way I kept Cam hydrated was to syringe or squirt milk into his mouth.

We stayed in hospital for four days under supposed 'observation', but other than getting Cam's tongue-tie snipped (see page 55) we received no further medical help or advice.

Obviously, due to my experience, I was fairly certain that

reflux was causing the problems (and because of my suspicions I had already ordered a breathing monitor for his cot) but, apart from one nurse, no medic would listen to or agree with me over the possible diagnosis. Upon discharge, however, Cameron was prescribed Infant Gaviscon* but given no further follow-up appointments and we were also signed off by the midwives.

Because of the feeding difficulties Cam experienced, it was impossible to log any feeds and sleeps during this time as, basically, there weren't any!

Did you know?

*Infant Gaviscon is a mild antacid that lines the oesophagus and negates some of the acid present in the digestive system. It is also designed to help thicken the feed when it combines with the gastic juices in the stomach. It is usually the first medication prescribed for infants who show signs of having reflux. See Chapter 7 on reflux for more information on this medication and on reflux itself.

Week 2

Hopefully you and baby are now home from hospital and settling into family life. You may still be under the care of a midwife, who will usually sign you off around Day 10. There are five checks that should be made before your midwife passes your care to a health visitor:

1.   Your baby has started to regain weight and is back to birth weight (see below).
2.   His umbilical cord has fallen off and the site is clean and dry.
3.   Any signs of jaundice have started to subside.
4.   He is feeding well and has no tongue-tie (see page 55).
5.   He is frequently having wet and dirty nappies.

Did you know?

Jaundice is caused by an excess of bilirubin in the baby's blood. Bilirubin is a yellow end-product of the normal breakdown of oxygen-carrying red blood cells and is usually removed from the bloodstream and processed by the liver, then passed into the kidneys to be expelled as urine. Many newborns produce more bilirubin than their immature livers can cope with and as a result it builds up in the blood, causing a yellow tinge to appear on the baby's body. This yellowing often starts at the head and works down, even colouring the whites of the eyes. This is relatively common in newborns and is known as physiological jaundice. It usually starts around Day 2 or 3 and should naturally subside by around Day 10. Natural sunlight and frequent fluid intake can help to break down and flush out the bilirubin from the baby's system.

Most babies will lose weight in the first few days and this is thought to be largely due to the passing of all the meconium that is in their intestines at birth (see pages 30 and 121). The guidelines are that there is usually an accepted loss of up to 10 per cent of birth weight, but any loss greater than this should be investigated. After around Day 3, weight should start to increase gradually and by the time your baby's care is passed over to the health visitor, he should have regained his original birth weight.

Your health visitor will give you a 'red book' which will chart all your baby's medical progress for the next five years. Within this book are weight and growth charts on which you can plot his development and keep a check on his weight over the weeks. The graphs record your baby's age and weight, which will set him on a centile in the graph. Head circumference and length should usually tally with the centile for weight; if there is a big difference between them there may need to be some medical investigation to find the cause. Your baby's weight should show a steady rise – essentially he should stay on or near his original birth centile. If his weight drops over two centiles on the graph, then you should seek some medical advice to find out why. See also Chapter 7 on reflux and feeding problems.

After his initial weight loss in the first few days, Cameron failed to regain any weight but slowly continued to lose and had already dropped over a centile on his weight graph by Day 10. However, with the introduction of the Infant Gaviscon and some formula to supplement feeding, his weight stabilized for a few days. On Day 12 we took him to London to see Dr Eltumi, a leading paediatric-gastro consultant, who confirmed my diagnosis of severe reflux and prescribed Nutramigen formula and Ranitidene and advised continuing the use of the Gaviscon. Things immediately calmed down, but although Cam was much better he still took ages to feed, was very windy and would often vomit.

We were now, though, able to start implementing 3-hourly feeds during the day and although some days started at 6am and others at 8am we could still get a quick bath and bedtime routine in place before the last feed of the day. Often, though, Cam would not settle to bed much before 9 or 10pm and we would have to give him another small feed before he would finally sleep. Sometimes he would then sleep through till the early hours, but on other nights he would wake during the late evening and then again in the early hours. We never knew what to expect – it was impossible to predict what each night would bring. Since Cam was born we had been swaddling him and sleeping him on alternate sides when he was put in his Moses basket, but by the end of this week we had resorted to sleeping him on his front as this was the only way he was comfortable enough ever to settle to sleep.

At this point, against my better judgement, we also had to introduce a dummy to help Cam settle. He was so uncomfortable and became so distressed that the only thing that helped was giving him a dummy to suck on. We tried to limit its use and where possible would settle him to sleep without it, but it soon became a crutch that not only Cameron relied on, but Chelsea as well. This is so very typical of babies with reflux, as they can still get comfort from sucking but without the discomfort of actually having to take milk.

Did you know?

Nutramigen formula is a specially designed formula for babies who are suffering from reflux and/or have any diet-related intolerance to cow's-milk protein and lactose.

Ranitidene is a medication prescribed by doctors for babies who are suffering from acid reflux.

For more information on all the above, see Chapter 7.

Cameron's journal: sixth and seventh days of Week 2 (Days 13 and 14 since birth)

Day	Feed	Amount	Nappy	Sleep	Comment
6	1.30am	80ml	W/D		Back asleep by 2.30am.
	5.30am	60ml	W/D		Slept till 8.15am.
	9am	50ml	W/D		Settled at 10am.
	11.55am	65ml	W/D		
	3.30pm	35ml	W		Screaming and crying, very unhappy . . . so am I!!
	7pm	65ml	W		Wouldn't settle for sleep so slept on Mummy!
7	12.45am	80ml	W/D		Settled in bed at 2am.
	5.15am	70ml	W		
	8am	60ml	W/D		Very slow feed . . . this takes ages?

Day	Feed	Amount	Nappy	Sleep	Comment	(cont.)
7	11am	60ml	W		Slept well in pram.	
	2pm	60ml	W/D		Slept on my chest.	
	4.45pm	50ml	W		Took an hour to feed.	
	8pm	80ml	W		Didn't settle to bed.	
	10.20pm	50ml	W/D		Finally got him settled by midnight . . . help, I don't want to do this any more!	

Week 3

By now the newest member of your family will have made his presence well and truly felt. Relatives will be eager to meet him and if you have other children the realization that baby is here to stay will have started to sink in! There is much advice available on how to prepare your toddler and/or older children for the new arrival, but nothing can ever truly ready them for the reality that hits as your new baby demands so much of Mummy's time and attention.

Many women today are having children much closer together as they choose to start their families comparatively late in life. It is very common these days for mothers to be coping with two children under the age of two and often three under the age of four. The main problem, I have found, is that many mothers struggle to deal with the whole bath and bedtime routine at the end of the day when they have a toddler or two to cope with as well as a new baby. Many find it easier initially to concentrate on the older children and see to the baby when the others are in bed asleep. However, the new baby can quickly learn that one-to-one time with Mummy and/or Daddy occurs later in the evening and he may then be reluctant to settle in bed at all. It can be really difficult to try to juggle this time of day when you have a new baby and older children to look after, but I urge you to try to stick to my plan with your newborn as much as possible if you want to avoid any sleep problems further down the line.

Mum's the Word . . .

I've now had three boys and followed Alison's plan with all of them. I have learned that it doesn't matter if things don't always seem to go smoothly, but if you just keep going you and your baby will get there in the end. My eldest and youngest boys slept through the night by about Week 7, but my middle baby had a few more problems and took longer – until Week 12 – to achieve the 12 hours. Bathtime was often quite a struggle but I always made sure to keep bedtime in place for them all . . . and it worked. All my boys still happily go to bed and sleep through the night . . . thanks, Alison!

G. C.

Moving into Week 3 Cameron was, on the whole, feeding on schedule and having five feeds during the day and two at night. However, the evenings were sometimes still a problem and he insisted on having an extra top-up feed at around 9 or 10pm. On Day 16 he fed at 7.15am, 10am, 1pm, 4pm, 7pm, 9pm and 11.15pm. He then slept through the night till 6.30am and the note in Chelsea's diary says, 'I was really worried as he didn't wake in the night and although he stirred a little at 6am he has not cried for food yet – Help, Mum, is he OK?' The next night he reverted to normal and fed at 10.50pm and 2.50am, then went through till 6.30am. So although the nights were still very erratic, the days were usually better and he enjoyed his 3-hourly feeding pattern.

Cameron's journal: second and third days of Week 3 (Days 16 and 17 since birth)

Day	Feed	Amount	Nappy	Sleep	Comment
2	3.45am	85ml	W/D		Asleep by 4.30am.
	8.15am	85ml	W		Only 1 hour's sleep.
	11.30am	60ml	W		Not good feed.
	1.30pm	55ml	W/D		Very slow feed but then slept well.
	4.50pm	60ml	W		Quite agitated and needed lots of cuddles.
	7.30pm	60ml	W/D		Settled by 8.50pm.
	10.10pm	60ml	W		Wouldn't settle again till 12.30am! I am tired!!!
3	3.55am	70ml	W		Settled by 4.20am.
	7.15am	70ml	W/D		Good sleep.
	10am	60ml	W/D		
	1pm	70ml	W/D		Slept in car on way to be registered!
	4pm	75ml	W/D		Didn't sleep much.
	7pm	70ml	W		Settled by 8pm.

Day	Feed	Amount	Nappy	Sleep	Comment	(cont.)
3	9pm	80ml			Fed well but will not settle so gave dummy.	
	11.15pm	40ml	W		Vomited and finally settled by 1am but then slept through till 6.15am!!!!!	

Week 4

At this stage you should see a regular daily pattern of feeds and sleeps begin to emerge, with your baby starting to sleep for longer after going to bed and not waking for his first night feed much before 1am.

If for any reason your baby was born more than two weeks prematurely, it is difficult to say at what stage he will be able to follow this plan and sleep for longer stretches, as he may need a week or two to catch up. I recently worked with a baby girl who was born at thirty weeks and came home from hospital five weeks later. I became involved in her care when she was eight weeks old from birth, which is minus two weeks corrected age (i.e. still two weeks before her due date). She was able to follow my plan relatively easily and by Week 13 from birth, which was three weeks old corrected age, she was sleeping 12 hours through each night. Most premature babies will be able to follow this plan: it is just a question of starting on the 3-hourly feeding schedule as soon as possible and leaving them to sleep at night once you have medical clearance that they no longer have to be woken for round-the-clock feeds.

> Things carried on pretty much the same during this week, with Cameron still having two feeds during the night. However, the evenings had settled down somewhat and more often than not we were able to get him settled in bed by 8pm. Chelsea was finding things really tough, though, as feeds could easily take up to an hour and Cameron still suffered with a lot of wind and frequently vomited. However, on the whole he was doing OK, was more alert and his weight had started slowly creeping up.

Cameron's journal: second and third days of Week 4 (Days 23 and 24 since birth)

Day	Feed	Amount	Nappy	Sleep	Comment
2	3.10am	100ml	W/D		Settled by 4.10am.
	7.10am	55ml	W	8.30am	Slept 1½ hours.
	10.10am	80ml	W/D		
	12.45pm	45ml	W		Not interested in feed, slept 2 hours.
	3.45pm	115ml	W/D		Had time awake, very happy!
	6.45pm	90ml	W		Asleep by 7.30pm.
	9.50pm	60ml	W		Settled by 10.50pm.
3	2.20am	80ml	W		Asleep by 3.10am.
	7.15am	110ml	W	8.30am	Good 1½-hour sleep.
	10.30am	80ml	W/D		
	1pm	90ml	W		Good feed and good sleep.
	3.55pm	55ml	W/D		Fed OK.
	7.15pm	85ml	W		
	10.20pm	70ml	W		Settled by 11.45pm.

Week 5

Moving into Week 5, your baby should be starting to sleep through into the early hours before waking for his one and only night feed. It may mean that he is waking at 6am ready for his first feed, which can seem to be a very early start to the day, but do persevere with following the plan as it will not be for ever and this stage will soon pass.

Many parents with twins or triplets have contacted me over the years to ask for a routine that they can use for their babies. My advice is always the same: follow my Sensational Baby Sleep Plan as it not only works for just one baby but for two and even three! In fact, one of the first articles that I had published was a case study on a set of triplets with whom I worked in 2002. They were born at 36 weeks and I implemented my plan from the start. At each feed mum would breastfeed one of the babies and I would feed the other two with bottles. They all shared one bedroom – in fact they all slept together in a cot-bed for the first five weeks – and by the time they were five weeks old corrected age (nine weeks from birth) they were all sleeping 11–12 hours each night. The key to making this plan work for multiples is to feed them all at the same time rather than staggering the feed times, which would mean that you have little or no time for anything else at all during the day as you would spend all your time feeding the babies. The other fundamental difference is that, when one baby wakes at night for a feed, it is best to wake the other(s) and feed them together so that they stay on the same schedule.

'How', I hear you shout, 'are you supposed to feed two, let alone three, babies at the same time?' Well, it does come with practice and it depends whether you are breast- or bottlefeeding. Some women can manage fairly well to breastfeed twins at the same time once they get the hang of it, but it is a slightly more difficult prospect if you have triplets! The answer is to enlist as much help as possible and ask someone else to feed at least one baby while you feed the other(s) at the breast. During the night it may be easier to bottlefeed all the babies, as this is often more manageable than breastfeeding when they are small. Sit on a large sofa or double bed, prop the babies up on soft but supportive pillows in front of you and use little beanbags to prop their bottles in place so they can feed. Some mums find that using rocking chairs or specially designed feeding beanbags can be a big help.

Usually I advise sleeping twins and triplets together at the start, separating them only if you find that they really start to disturb each other. However, unless there is any degree of reflux or digestive discomfort that prevents them from sleeping comfortably, I have generally found that they will sleep perfectly well in the same room.

Mum's the Word . . .

Alison was the main reason that our twins started sleeping through. I was in too much shock to be capable of getting them into a routine. Alison immediately put them on her 3-hourly feeding routine and I believe that if it had not been for her help they would have been awake at all hours for months. Under her guidance, I was amazed how easy I soon found being able to feed both babies together. She also gave us the confidence to put them in their own room and within weeks they were sleeping 12 hours each night.

D. L.

By the middle of Week 5 Cameron was settling much better in the evening and was generally in bed and asleep by around 7.30pm. He had also started to wake only once in the night for a feed, usually anywhere between midnight and 2am. He was then waking around 6.30am for his first daytime feed. He was still on the 3-hourly feeding plan during the day and was still having Nutramigen formula, Ranitidine three times a day and a sachet of Infant Gaviscon in each feed. His weight was slowly going up and he was averaging up to 600ml of feed in each 24 hours, which meant he was taking six feeds of around 100ml each time. This isn't a huge volume for a five-week-old baby, but we were happy as there was some weight gain and he was more settled than in previous weeks.

Cameron's journal: third and sixth days of Week 5 (Days 31 and 34 since birth)

Day	Feed	Amount	Nappy	Sleep	Comment
3	3.20am	100ml	W/D		Settled by 4.15am.
	7.20am	80ml	W	9am	Slept for an hour.
	10.30am	110ml	W/D		Refused to sleep at all.
	12.45pm	60ml	W		Not good feed, he was tired! Then slept 2½ hours!
	3.50pm	110ml	W		
	6.50pm	120ml	W		Settled by 8pm.
6	1.10am	100ml	W/D		Settled by 2am.
	6.30am	125ml	W	8am	Slept only 45 mins.
	10.15am	100ml	W	11am	Slept for 90 mins.
	12.55pm	80ml	W		Fed well.
	4pm	80ml	W/D		Large vomit, not good feed.
	6.50pm	110ml	W		Settled by 7.35pm.

Week 6

Life should be a little more settled for you and your baby by now and with any luck you will be feeling more confident about how to adapt the plan on a daily basis so that you are able to get out and about on most days. With your baby still being on 3-hourly feeds it can be quite an art to juggle feed and sleep times to allow you time outside the house, but if you try to plan your outings around feed times it will make life easier. For instance, if you want to go out in the morning you can either give Feed 2 before you go out and let your baby sleep in the pram or the car, then give Feed 3 when you get back; or go out before Feed 2 and take it with you to offer en route; or dash out quickly between the two feeds.

If you need to go out in the evening and don't have a babysitter, I suggest that you do your normal bath and bedtime routine, give your baby his last feed and put him to 'bed' either in his car seat, carrycot or pram, depending on where you are going and how you are getting there. Hopefully he will sleep while you are out and then when you get home you can transfer him into his cot. If he seems unsettled by being moved from pram to cot, then re-settle him with a quick feed, but only if really necessary.

> After having such a good week, it seemed that Cam 'regressed' slightly as we moved into Week 6. He had a couple of nights where he woke two or three times and needed an extra feed, and his feeds were really difficult during the day. But by the end of the week things seemed to have settled again and he was back to just one feed during the night at around 3am.

Alison says . . .

Of course, this is typical of a reflux baby because when they have a good week and eat and sleep well, they then have a growth spurt and 'outgrow' the sphincter muscle and valve, and the reflux symptoms seem temporarily to come back with a vengeance!

Cameron's journal: first and seventh days of Week 6 (Days 36 and 42 since birth)

Day	Feed	Amount	Nappy	Sleep	Comment
1	1.20am	145ml	W		Vomited and took ages to settle.
	6.50am	100ml	W	8.50am	Took ages to go back to sleep for nap.
	10.05am	90ml	W/D	11am	Asleep for nap and slept 90 mins.
	1pm	150ml	W		Vomited a lot of feed.
	3.50pm	100ml	W		Seemed very windy and took ages over feed.
	6.40pm	110ml	W		Not a good feed, cried throughout. Hungry? Tired? In pain? I don't know!! Very difficult to settle.
7	1.30am	85ml	W/D		Settled back to bed by 2.40am.
	7am	140ml	W/D		Woke at 6.30am, but dozed on and off till 7am.
	10.05am	90ml	W		Feed took an hour and a half!
	1.30pm	80ml	W		
	4.05pm	65ml	W		Useless feed, Cam just gets to a point and refuses!
	6.45pm	145ml	W		Settled and asleep by 8pm after a better feed.

Week 7

Statistics suggest that the majority of mothers give up breastfeeding around this stage. Although there are many different reasons for this, I believe that it is in part due to the lack of help and support available, but mainly because of the guidelines that suggest it is best for your baby if you exclusively breastfeed for six months. Rather than feeling under so much pressure, mothers should be encouraged to take a more relaxed approach to feeding. If they received support in introducing a supplementary feed as necessary – as my feeding guide suggests – I believe many would continue breastfeeding for longer. Surely if a baby receives at least some breast milk each day it is better than none at all?

If you have reached this point and do want to give up breastfeeding, see Chapter 2, pages 49–54 for advice on how best to achieve this.

By now your daytime feeds should be forming much more of a pattern and there should be just the one feed at night. If you are still really struggling and your baby does not seem to be responding to the feed and sleep schedule at all, then I advise you to read Chapter 7 and try to discover why he is unable to follow this plan. There is nearly always an underlying reason and it is often due to a digestive problem of some description, related to milk intolerances, allergies or reflux.

> Although Cameron's daytime feeds were regular and well established, he was still taking a very long time to finish his milk and his intake was still on the low side. He was sleeping much better at night and going to bed more easily, but was still often disturbed by wind during his sleeps, whether it was during the day or night, and we would have to re-settle him, often with a dummy. However, during this week he woke only during two nights for a feed; on the others he actually slept through from bedtime till morning!

Alison says . . .

Although Cam's milk intake was a little low, because he was still managing a small weight increase each week my advice to Chelsea was not to wake him at night just to get a little more milk into him. In my experience a really good sleep will be more beneficial to a baby than a couple of extra ounces of milk. Once a baby is sleeping well and more rested, it will often have the knock-on effect of improving feed intake.

Cameron's journal: second and fifth days of Week 7 (Days 44 and 47 since birth)

Day	Feed	Amount	Nappy	Sleep	Comment
2					Woke at 2.10am, just gave water and then dummy.
	6.45am	100ml	W	8am	Sleep back in bed for 1¼ hours.
	10.05am	120ml	W/D		Refused to sleep!
	1.40pm	60ml	W/D		
	4.50pm	70ml	W		Very tired!! I am not surprised, Cam!!!
	7.40pm	110ml	W/D		Settled and asleep by 8.40pm.
5					Slept through the night without stirring!
	7am	140ml	W/D	9am	Sleep for 1 hour.

Day	Feed	Amount	Nappy	Sleep	Comment	(cont.)
1	10.30pm	115ml	W		Sleep for 45 mins.	
	1.15pm	90ml	W/D		Slept in pram.	
	3.45pm	95ml	W			
	7pm	140ml	W/D		Settled after much winding by 8.30pm.	

Week 8

By this stage your baby should be showing signs that he really doesn't need a feed during the night. If he is still waking in the early hours and looking for his feed, this might be the time to think about watering it down – see pages 105 and 112 – and offering a less concentrated feed. It is often the case that a baby who still insists on having a feed around 3 or 4am is not then really interested in his first feed in the morning . Watering down the night feed will therefore encourage him to take his milk at Feed 1 rather than during the night.

By now, most babies who have reached 4.10kg (9lb) in weight are capable of sustaining a 12-hour period throughout the night without the need for food.

Being woken up in the early hours of the morning can be very tiring and I am sure it is from this situation that the so-called 'dream feed' was devised and advised by many other babycare experts. The thinking is that it is easier for parents to give their baby a feed at 10 or 11pm before they go to bed in the hope that the baby will have a long period of sleep from 11pm through to 6 or 7am, allowing them to get a chunk of sleep. However, this is designed to meet the needs of the parents and not the needs of the baby, and, as we have seen, it can actually have a detrimental effect on the baby's developing sleep pattern.

Following my plan, undoubtedly there will be a few weeks where you have to get up during the early hours to give your baby a feed, but this doesn't last for long and soon your baby will be sleeping through the night.

> At the beginning of this week Cameron's reflux medication was changed and Dr Eltumi prescribed Losec Mups in the hope that it would help him feed more comfortably.
>
> Cam was sometimes still waking anywhere between 2 and 5am and wanting a feed, but was then not interested in his first feed of the day. I advised that Chelsea start to water down and reduce the volume of the feed she offered in the early hours, and by the end of the week he was taking just a small drink of water and feeding properly at 7am instead.
>
> This was still a tough week. Cam was quite unsettled a lot of the time, although as the Losec started to kick in we did begin to see a gradual improvement by the end of the week.

Did you know?

Losec is a more effective medication in the treatment of acid reflux and is often prescribed by a paediatrician to help reduce the acid levels in a baby's digestive system. See Chapter 7 on reflux, which explains the use of this drug in more detail.

Cameron's journal: first and fifth days of Week 8 (Days 50 and 54 since birth)

Day	Feed	Amount	Nappy	Sleep	Comment
1					Woke at 1.30am, cried for a few minutes then went back to sleep.
	6.55am	170ml	W/D	8.15am	Slept for 90 mins.
	10am	120ml	W		Refused to sleep.

Day	Feed	Amount	Nappy	Sleep	Comment	(cont.)
1	12.50pm	110ml	W/D	1.45pm	Slept for 90 mins.	
	3.40pm	130ml	W			
	6.30pm	125ml	W		Settled by 7.30pm.	
5					Woke at 12.50, gave water.	
	6.50pm	150ml	W/D	9am	Struggled to settle for sleep and woke after 45 mins.	
	10.40pm	140ml	W	11am	Still not sleeping well . . . absolute nightmare!	
	1.15am	140ml	W		Large vomit. Will only cat-nap.	
	4pm	100ml	W/D	4.30pm	Finally slept 1 hour.	
	6.45pm	110ml	W		Settled by 7.45pm.	

Week 9

Having just started to eradicate the last night feed, you might think it is too soon to start dropping a daytime feed as well. However, as in Cameron's case, some babies will respond quite readily to dropping from five to four feeds during the day at this point and it can often have a positive impact not only on their intake of feed but on their night sleep as well. For some babies, especially those with reflux, the advice is to feed little and often, but this can actually cause more problems than it resolves. Many seem to do better with longer gaps between feeds and actually take more milk at each feed when put on to a 4-hourly schedule. As a result, their total daily intake increases and they then sleep better at night. See Chapter 4 on how to implement the Sensational Baby Sleep Plan to find out more about dropping a daytime feed.

This is a typical situation in which you will need to trust your instincts and judge for yourself whether your baby is ready to drop a feed during the day or whether he is still quite happy to stay on his 3-hourly schedule for another few weeks. If the latter is the case, I would advise that you do change to the 4-hourly schedule sometime before your baby is three months old.

> Having been on Losec for over a week now, things had really begun to improve for Cameron. We decided to drop to 4-hourly feeds in the hope that it would increase his intake and this actually worked beautifully. His feed levels went up and therefore his total daily intake increased to an average of 700ml.
>
> He also started to sleep through the night properly without any disturbances except the odd 'wake and whinge' around 5am from which he would settle himself back to sleep.
>
> I also believe Cam's night sleeping improved because, with the introduction of Losec, Chelsea was able to see that he was no longer in so much discomfort. This meant she felt able to leave him a little longer to settle himself to sleep without rushing to comfort him in the way that, understandably, she had been doing up to now. In fact, under my guidance, when Cam wouldn't settle at bedtime she would reassure him through the two-way monitor and was amazed at how quickly this worked in settling him down to sleep.

Cameron's journal: second and sixth days of Week 9 (Days 58 and 62 since birth)

Day	Feed	Amount	Nappy	Sleep	Comment
2					Woke at 5am, reassurance through monitor and went back to sleep.
	6.45am	160ml	W/D	8.30am	Would only sleep for an hour.

Day	Feed	Amount	Nappy	Sleep	Comment	(cont.)
2	10.30am	145ml	W	11.30am	Slept well for 2 hours.	
	2.30pm	145ml	W/D		Well, alert and happy.	
	6.15pm	180ml	W		Settled (still with dummy) at 7.45pm.	
6					Slept through.	
	6.10am	180ml	W/D	8.15am	Slept 90 mins.	
	10.20am	160ml	W	11am	Slept in pram 1 hour.	
	2.10pm	180ml	W/D		Reasonable afternoon.	
	6.30pm	180ml	W		Still not settled till 8pm.	

Week 10

As you can see from Cameron's story, it is so easy – and sometimes necessary – to slip into the habit of using a pacifier or dummy. It is not something that I generally advise, but I am very aware that the reality of looking after a new baby is that sometimes you just have to do whatever is necessary to get through from one day to the next. However, as with Cam, there will usually come a time when you need to persuade your baby to stop using the dummy as it often starts to create more sleep problems than it resolves. The quickest way to stop is to choose a suitable day and then simply put (or throw) away all the dummies you have in circulation. You may decide to choose a day when you are quite busy and hope the distraction of lots going on will help the baby to forget that he is missing his dummy, or you may prefer to have a couple of days at home in order to have more time to help him re-adjust. You will also find it helpful to read Chapter 6, which explains how to use my reassurance sleep-training technique and where you will find some good advice on how to settle your baby without using a dummy.

Up until now, although Cameron had been following the plan relatively well, we still sometimes had a problem with settling him to sleep, especially for daytime naps. I realized that the time had come to remove his dummy completely and after explaining the reasons to Chelsea she agreed to give it a go. It was a really difficult decision on her part, because she admitted that she felt totally 'freaked' whenever Cam cried and at least she knew that by giving him his dummy he would generally stop crying – even though he still might not settle to sleep but just keep wanting the dummy replaced! However, after just one day without it, Cam seemed to forget that he had ever had a dummy and, although things were still far from ideal with his daytime sleeps, generally he was starting to settle more easily.

Chelsea then explained to me how she felt about taking Cam out without his dummy. She hated him crying in front of other people when they were out, and without the dummy she was terrified of being unable to stop him crying. It took longer for her to come to terms with this than it did for Cam to adapt to life without his dummy: the issue was much more about building her confidence as a mum.

Alison says . . .

We have all been guilty of looking or staring when we hear a baby cry or a toddler throw a tantrum in public. Even though we may actually feel sorry for the parent, the looks do nothing but make them wish the ground would open up and swallow them.

Cameron's journal: second and fifth days of Week 10 (Days 65 and 68 since birth)

Day	Feed	Amount	Nappy	Sleep	Comment
2					Stirred at 4.30 and 5.55am but settled by himself without the dummy!
	6.35am	180ml	W/D	8.15am	Back to bed, slept OK without dummy.
	10.15am	175ml	W	noon	Fed OK but sleepy, put to bed at 12, slept 2 hours.
	2.55pm	175ml	W/D		
	6.15pm	175ml	W		Settled to sleep at 7.50pm without dummy!
5					Slept through, no stirrings . . . hooray!
	6.30am	180ml	W/D	8.30am	First nap of 90 mins.
	10.15am	180ml	W	12.30pm	Slept 1 hour then didn't go back to sleep!
	2.15pm	180ml	W		
	6.20pm	180ml	W		Settled by 7.40pm.

Week 11

If you haven't already done so, it would be a good idea to make plans for dropping from 3-hourly to 4-hourly feeds as explained in Chapter 4 on page 115. Also, if your baby is still resisting to giving up his last night feed, I would advise that you water it down for a few days and then offer only water at night. See Chapter 6, which explains how to settle your baby once you have removed the last night feed.

As happened with Cameron, the final things to fall into place when following this plan are often the daytime sleeps. Many babies need a little extra encouragement before they will readily accept them. I find that the sleeps are easier to achieve once your baby is on the 4-hourly schedule than in the early weeks when the 3-hourly feeding schedule is in place and there is less time for sleeping between feeds. Again, see Chapter 6 on how best to establish daytime naps if you are experiencing any problems.

It all seems such a breeze now – Cameron is feeding and gaining weight at an astonishing rate. He actually put on 680g (1½ lb) in two weeks and is sleeping 11–12 hours each night without waking up at all. However, the hardest part of this week was to help Chelsea carry out some sleep-training for daytime naps. Luckily Cam responded very quickly and it was all soon a memory! Cam still has odd days that are quite difficult, but on the whole his reflux seems to be stable, for the time being at least, and we are due to visit Dr Eltumi soon for a review.

During the early weeks I'm not so sure that Chelsea believed in my plan and really found it tough to stick to the 3-hourly feeds. But now that Cameron is sleeping through the night (unlike the babies of her friends who have not followed this plan) she, like many of my clients before her, is now one of the Sensational Baby Sleep Plan's biggest fans!

Although Chelsea continued to keep a diary and chart for six months, there is no need to put any further excerpts in at this stage as Cameron was regularly taking four feeds each day at around 7am, 11am, 2.30pm and 6.30pm and sleeping through the night.

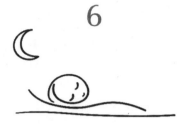

6

The Reassurance
Sleep-training Technique

This chapter is aimed at parents with babies aged three to four months and over who have not followed my Sensational Baby Sleep Plan from the early weeks and whose babies may therefore not yet be sleeping through the night or having structured daytime sleeps. It is also important for parents who have followed the plan to understand how to use this technique if their babies unexpectedly stop sleeping well during the day or start waking at night. This may be caused by a bout of illness or teething, moving house or travelling away from home, or by any other disruption to normal daily life.

I have come across and read about many methods of sleep-training, ranging from strict controlled crying to a 'no-cry' sleep solution. Having mixed a few points from various methods with my own knowledge and understanding of babies and their sleep habits, I have devised what I call the 'reassurance sleep-training technique'.

More often than not, the families with whom I have worked have already tried many sleep-training methods without success, devised some of their own and introduced countless other so-called sleep aids. As desperation sets in, parents can suddenly find themselves carrying out utterly crazy rituals just to get a couple of hours' sleep. The following are just a few examples of situations that I have encountered:

○ Lying awake next to a baby in order to replace his dummy as soon as he stirs.
○ Parents doing shifts to sit up through the night rocking their baby to sleep in their arms.
○ Having a buggy in the baby's room and walking him round and round throughout the night to keep him asleep.
○ Still swaddling a baby of seven months to try to give him security.
○ Giving the baby sleep-inducing medication on a nightly basis.
○ Pushing their baby in his pushchair or driving him in the car around the streets in the middle of the night.
○ Leaving as many as *six* full bottles of milk for an older baby to find for himself and drink throughout the night.
○ Commonly, parents sleeping in separate rooms so that one can sleep while the other stays awake trying to settle the baby throughout the

night. (This may be useful in the early weeks while night feeds are still necessary, but should not need to be a long-term solution.)

○ One mother, desperately wanting to get her ten-month-old out of the marital bed, achieved this by climbing into the cot with the baby to get him to sleep. She would then climb out when he was asleep, but climb back in during the night when he woke so that she could re-settle him. This mum called me for help the morning after the cot had broken!

In these and similar scenarios, I am happy to say that all the parents do look back and are able to have a good laugh at the crazy situations in which they found themselves. Of course this does not detract from the agonizing, sleep deprivation and the sheer desperation that drove them to such extremes at the time.

At the same time, it is very important for you not to blame yourself. I always say to parents that it matters not why or how you have ended up in the situation you are in: it has always arisen from circumstances. Maybe you were afraid that your new baby would disturb and wake your toddler if you allowed him to cry at all during the night, so you introduced a number of soothing techniques to keep the baby from crying. It may be that you were unaware that your baby was suffering from reflux and before you had a diagnosis the only way you could get him to sleep was by holding him upright on your chest with a dummy. Or perhaps you were following another babycare method and were demand feeding throughout the night or offering a dream feed that your baby is now reluctant to give up? There are so many reasons that may have led to you and your baby suffering from sleep deprivation (see Chapters 1 and 3), but in nearly all cases none was intentional on your part. No parent has ever *set out* to have a baby who doesn't sleep through the night, the parent ending up so exhausted that they struggle to function. This has always come from one of the classic 'accidental parenting' situations.

So every parent will benefit from understanding how to use my reassurance sleep-training technique. Even if you have followed my plan from Day 1 and your baby sleeps through the night, there are many variables that can cause changes in our normal daily pattern, easily upsetting a baby's routine and possibly causing him to start waking at night. As you will discover later in this chapter, a baby will easily forget a learned habit or association, but equally he will learn a new one just as quickly. It is therefore vital that you know how to deal with any night-waking as soon as it occurs, thus avoiding the formation of any negative, long-term sleep habits.

I have helped hundreds of families resolve sleep problems with babies who range in age from three months to two years. My reassurance sleep-training technique, with just a few age-sensitive adaptations and appropriate adjustments for the individual, has proved to be 100 per cent successful.

Mum's the Word . . .

My twins were nine months old when Alison came to stay with us. Neither of them had slept a night through and as the babies got older the situation had deteriorated with, at worst, Nicolai waking every few hours and not settling for hours at a time even though he was in our bed. I had even resorted to separating the twins, and as neither would settle in their cots in the nursery I kept one baby at home who slept in our bed while the other would spend the nights with my parents in their bed. Also, as we had no daytime routine with the boys at all, and with my lively two-year-old to cope with too, we were all at breaking point. I couldn't see how we were ever going to survive the situation, we were all so tired.

I had expected Alison to stay with us for up to a week to help with the babies' sleeping but within one night after implementing her sleep-training routine she had fixed the problem. On Night 2 both my boys slept without a sound and this continued on Night 3 and has done so since. Alison also helped put the boys into a fantastic daytime routine which they love – they are so happy to go into their cots for their daytime naps. They are now happy, well-rested, super-contented babies. Every mother's dream!

Although I desperately wanted the situation to change and get better I was still really anxious about 'sleep-training' as the phrase sounds quite harsh, but Alison's technique is wonderful. The babies are constantly reassured, which, in turn, made me feel able to see it through. The boys responded so well and were not distressed at all – it was truly remarkable to witness.

J. Z.

The effect of sleep deprivation on babies

Very few people realize that a baby can actually suffer from sleep deprivation and they do not understand why, if their baby is tired, he still refuses to sleep. The fact is, as explained in earlier chapters, we actually have to teach a baby to sleep by providing the right environment, differentiating between day and night, establishing a basic daily routine with a regular sequence of naps, and giving him the space and independence to develop a healthy sleep association. Over many years I have witnessed a lot of different behavioural displays that are the result of a baby being overtired.

Alison says . . .

Sleep deprivation is an internationally recognized form of torture, but few people realize what damaging effects a lack of sleep can have on themselves and their baby.

Some of the symptoms that an overtired baby may show are:

- appearing to be hyperactive or seeming not to need much sleep
- clawing at his face or scratching himself through frustration
- crying inconsolably for long periods
- having complete 'meltdowns', becoming apoplectic at times, or just seeming to 'lose it' completely

○   refusing feeds or taking only very small amounts
○   having no interest in the introduction of solid food
○   being quite miserable and fractious most of the time
○   rarely smiling or interacting
○   and rarely sleeping!

Mum's the Word . . .

My seven-month-old baby was waking about four times every night and each time I would try to re-settle him using either a feed, a dummy or both. Also, for two months I had been trying to get him to take some solids but he point blank refused and had never eaten any of it. I was at the point of thinking that he couldn't actually swallow anything but milk.

After contacting Alison I followed her advice and carried out her reassurance sleep-training. By Night 3 he had woken just once and was also taking proper naps during the day. The most amazing thing was that on Day 4 he suddenly began to eat his solids, I couldn't believe it! Alison had said that when he started to sleep properly, hopefully he would start to eat properly – and he did! I never thought that his being overtired would have caused him to refuse solids.

H. Y.

In many cases the parents are convinced that there is really something seriously wrong with their baby and do not link the symptoms with just a lack of sleep. This is not surprising, as some of the behaviour displayed can be quite extreme and, as I have already mentioned, you would think that if it was simply that the baby was tired then surely he would just sleep? However, this is just not the case. The problem is that, because his system is not getting the rest and sleep it actually needs, his body produces more and more adrenaline to keep it going, which in turn is not conducive to being able to fall into calm and restful sleep. In fact, the baby's system becomes so 'wired' that it just can't relax into sleep and the situation carries on in a downward spiral of being overtired, producing more adrenaline to survive and therefore not being able to relax into sleep.

Through my work I have come to realize that sleep deprivation in babies can have a far-reaching effect on their behaviour not only during infancy but also as they grow older. (Again, see Chapters 1 and 3 for more information on sleep and sleep deprivation.) In researching the behaviour displayed by children diagnosed with Attention Deficit Hyperactivity Disorder (ADHD), I have found great similarities to that displayed by babies suffering from severe sleep deprivation. I am able to trace a connection between babies who never learned to sleep well, showing at times some or all of the symptoms mentioned above, and their continuing poor sleep patterns and subsequent hyperactive behaviour as they get older. ADHD can be a very distressing disorder to cope with. I do not mean to make light of it in any way, nor to suggest that the sole cause is lack of sleep, but I firmly believe there is a very strong link between the two and there is indeed evidence that many children diagnosed with ADHD are also sleep deprived.[7] In fact, there is research-based evidence which states that sleep deprivation may cause permanent behavioural problems in children. It has been shown that many of these children have never slept well as babies and then continue to suffer with sleep problems as they get older.

Many parents, although they undoubtedly love their babies, can lose all ability to cope with simple day-to-day tasks when suffering from a severe lack of sleep. A further point to take into consideration here is that, if sleep deprivation has this detrimental effect on you, then it is highly likely that your baby is feeling the same way too!

How and why sleep problems can occur

There are many different reasons why a baby may not have learned to sleep through, or, having done so for some time, has now started to wake during the night.

○   My feeding and sleeping plan may not have been used within the
     first few weeks and therefore the baby may not have learned to sleep.

○ As also explained in Chapters 1 and 3, if you are not following any sort of daytime routine it is unlikely that your baby will be getting enough sleep, by way of structured naps during the day. This can then cause him to have a more disturbed night.

○ Generally your baby may have good structured daytime sleeps, but occasionally you may spend a whole day away from home when he is unable to take his naps so easily. This may have the knock-on effect of his having a disturbed night.

○ It might have been your choice to co-sleep with your baby in the early weeks, but you now find that he won't settle in his own bed.

○ Overanxious parents can unwittingly continually disturb their baby by constantly going into his room to check on him.

○ You may have been giving a dream feed after which your baby used to sleep through till the morning, but he is now waking several times each night.

○ Or perhaps you have tried to stop giving the dream feed but your baby is still waking and looking for it.

○ It may be time to introduce solids as your baby is waking at night due to hunger.

○ It may be that your baby was never able to sleep for long periods or could not settle to sleep easily due to being uncomfortable with digestive problems, dietary intolerances and/or gastric reflux. See Chapter 7 for information on this.

○ Some babies can have adverse reactions to their regular immunizations and may wake in the night feeling unwell.

○ Some babies can be disturbed through the onset of teething, especially if they cut a few teeth at an early age. This may cause them to wake at night and you may be finding it hard to re-settle them.

○ At some point your baby will probably get a cough or cold or have some other minor illness which may cause him to have a disturbed night and not sleep or settle easily.

○ The arrival of another baby can easily unsettle your toddler and may cause him to display some negative reactions, including waking at night.

○ Any change in your baby's usual environment, such as moving house, can cause him to be less settled at night.

○ Change in your family dynamics, such as dealing with a bereavement, a family split or any other stressful situation that life throws at you, may result in your baby or toddler picking up on the tense atmosphere and being generally more unsettled, especially at night.

○ Going to stay with friends and family, taking short breaks and staying in hotels, going on holiday, travelling abroad and encountering different time zones can all cause your baby to fall out of routine, suffer from disturbed nights and be unable to sleep as easily as when at home.

○ The hour change that occurs in the UK every March and October (see page 92 for more information on how to cope with this).

As you can see, there are many reasons why a baby may not have learned to sleep through or has suddenly started waking during the night. Whatever the cause, it can seem like a hopeless situation as, no matter what you have tried, nothing seems to help. Maybe you feel that your baby is the one for whom there is no sleep solution? Well, rest assured – nearly every parent who has asked for my help has felt that way and has been sure that their baby would be the one and only that would not respond to my reassurance sleep-training technique! Happily, they have all been wrong and although along the way some babies have certainly proved to be quite challenging, many more have responded with ease and surprised us all.

How and why the technique works

All babies learn by association and very quickly get used to repetitive patterns. One simple example is that you may have found it easier to settle your baby by taking him into bed with you, but within a matter of days this is what he will come to expect and so he will find it difficult to settle anywhere else. But the fact that babies will also learn new habits and forget the old just as quickly works in your favour when you start to implement my sleep-training method.

Another key point to understanding why this method works so well is that when you implement it you will be giving your baby one message and one message only, thus removing any previous confusion.

For instance, with such a wide variety of advice available to them many parents will have tried a multitude of different ways over a number of nights to try to get their baby to go to sleep: giving a feed, not giving a feed, using a dummy, leaving a light on, playing music, sitting by the cot and stroking his head, rocking him to sleep, leaving him to 'cry it out', sleeping next to him, trying him back in his cot, etc. – the list could go on for ever. All this can only lead to your baby feeling a little confused to say the least, and not really able to understand what is expected of him each night. 'Do I get cuddles or not?' 'Am I getting a feed tonight or not?' 'Do I get to sleep with Mummy and Daddy again?' 'I'm just not sure what is supposed to be happening at night . . . Help!' By using my reassurance sleep-training technique you will be able to eradicate all this confusion and reinforce one simple message: 'It's sleepy time!'

Another major factor contributing to my method's success is that it involves the removal of any existing negative sleep associations and the taking away of any sleep attachments that your baby has come to rely on. I hear you cry out in horror, but please don't be put off yet – just read on. It may seem like an absolute impossibility even to think of removing that dummy, but it can be done and your baby will sleep so much better after only a few nights. As I mentioned at the start of the book, among many of my clients I am known as the 'Magic Sleep Fairy' – but sadly, there is no 'sleepy dust', only my sleep-training method. Yes, there will be tears (often more from the parents than from the baby): your baby will cry at times, seem to be distressed or even angry, and he may well be. It's simple: babies do not like change and for a couple of days he will not understand why things have changed, but very quickly he will start to forget that he had Mummy's breast to go to sleep on or that he had his dummy being replaced ten times a night to comfort him. He will soon now begin to learn the new, more positive association of going to sleep in his cot, on his own and without any so-called sleep aids.

In fact, what you *and* your baby will very quickly begin to realize is that most of the things you were doing to try to help him sleep were actually more of a hindrance. This is because as a baby goes to sleep he will have a lasting impression of his surroundings and what was happening as he fell asleep. So when he then stirs during his sleep cycles, if things have changed it may upset or confuse him and cause to him to wake. For example, if he goes to sleep while suckling at your breast and you then put him into his cot already asleep, when he stirs he may well panic and wake up crying as his last memory is of being cuddled up with you and now he is alone in his cot. Whatever sleep aid you use to settle your baby, whether it is a dummy, rocking, a feed, stroking and patting him or anything else, he will then expect this every time he stirs throughout his natural sleep cycles. This is why my technique is the most effective way of teaching your baby to sleep. Although it may seem harsh to remove any sleep aids all at once, within two to three days your baby will have forgotten that they ever existed and he will be much more comfortable with and ready to accept his new sleep associations. Most parents are amazed at how quickly their baby adapts and settles so easily without all the previous sleep-associated rituals which had developed over time and become the norm.

Another contributing factor to the success of my method is that a change of the baby's sleep position can have a positive impact. As I have already explained in Chapters 1 and 3, throughout my experience I have found the majority of babies will sleep better and be far more comfortable on their side or even on their tummies.

Safety guidelines for implementing sleep-training

With many babies who do not sleep well there is often an underlying cause which needs to be addressed before tackling any form of sleep-training. A baby suffering from any digestive or dietary disorder such as reflux (see Chapter 7) will rarely be able to relax into sleep easily and may frequently be woken by pain or discomfort, therefore never learning to sleep for any length of time. You cannot expect a baby to sleep through the night if he is in any discomfort and it is very important to ensure that any possible reflux is properly diagnosed, treated and managed before carrying out sleep-training.

Always make sure that your baby is fit and well before embarking on my sleep-training. Any minor ailment could hinder the process, which would be unfair to both you and your baby. For instance, if he has a cold it would be better to wait a few days for the worst symptoms to pass so that he is feeling better in himself before introducing the changes you will be putting in place. Obviously some illnesses are not immediately apparent, but if you feel that your baby is more unsettled or cranky than usual it may be worth a trip to the GP to get him checked over, as he may have an ear infection or other hard-to-spot ailment. If your baby is taken ill soon after implementing sleep-training, try not to despair: although it may be a temporary setback, do read pages 93–4 and 194–5 on dealing with illness which will explain how to cope.

Teething can be an obvious cause of pain to any baby, but in my experience unless your baby has severe teething symptoms it should not hinder the sleep-training programme.

It is usually best to carry out my reassurance sleep-training programme at a time when you have a fairly free week or so in your diary, and try to ensure that it is not going to coincide with your baby's vaccinations.

Preparing for sleep-training

As well as taking into account the safety guidelines set out in the previous section, there are other factors of which you need to be aware because they can affect the success of this sleep-training technique:

○ It is essential that everyone involved with the care of your baby understands how to use the method, is fully committed to it and is also prepared to give you as much support as possible throughout the next few days and nights.
○ Everyone must follow the same pattern and reinforce the 'sleepy-time' message, because if just one person decides to pick your baby up for a cuddle when he is crying during sleep-training, it can cancel all the effort and progress made up to that point and you will have to start again.
○ If you are the only one in your household who wants to use the technique it can be very disheartening if, say, your partner is not helpful throughout the night, makes negative comments or even tries to do something different. It is so much easier if you are in total

agreement about using this method before trying to implement it as then you can support each other throughout the process.

○ However many times you may have previously tried, albeit unsuccessfully, to use other sleep-training methods, it is so important to find the strength and resolve to see this technique through. I appreciate it may be hard to find the faith and belief that this will work, but I can assure you that it does. Very quickly you will begin to see positive improvements in your baby's sleep, which in turn will give you the confidence to carry on.

○ The more times that you give up and try to re-start, the more difficult it will become because your baby will quickly learn that there is still no consistency from one night to the next.

○ When implementing this technique, the best results are achieved more quickly if your baby is in his own room. I realize that government guidelines advise you to have the baby in your room until he is at least six months old, but it is a simple fact that he, and you, usually sleep more soundly when he is in his own room. See Chapter 3 for more detailed information on the issue of where your baby should sleep. If space is not available and he has to stay in your room, move his cot to a quiet, dark corner as far away from your bed as possible. You may even put up a curtain or screen to partition off an area and so keep him as separate as possible from your sleeping area.

○ If your baby shares a room with an older sibling, then if possible, and just while you implement the technique, it might be helpful to move the older child to another room or even to stay with relatives or friends for a few nights. If, however, you have a toddler and a baby who share a room and neither of whom sleep well, it is possible to leave them in together and carry out the sleep-training for both at the same time. Likewise, if you have twins and they share a room it is fine to sleep-train them both together.

○ As I have explained in Chapter 3, I find many babies actually do not sleep well on their backs and it might assist the sleep-training process if you try them in different positions. Most can move around the cot by eight months anyway, and they will discover their own comfortable position in which to sleep. If you find your baby favours sleeping on his side or front, for your own peace of mind it is advisable to use an under-mattress breathing monitor (see pages 81–2).

○   It is not necessary to use total blackout blinds for the baby's room, but try to ensure there are curtains or a blind that provide a relatively good light shield.

○   It is not necessary to tiptoe around the house while your baby is actually asleep. All babies are used to the usual noise within their home environment and will learn to sleep through this. However, if, for example, someone in the family is learning to play the drums, it would be advisable for them not to practise during your baby's sleep times!

○   Try to set aside a couple of weeks when your diary is relatively free and you are able to stay at home most days so that you can focus on the whole sleep-training process.

○   For a few nights prior to starting sleep-training it can be helpful to keep a diary of your baby's sleep, or the lack of it, during both the day and the night (see page 114). Continuing with the sleep diary throughout the whole process is a useful way of charting your baby's progress, and you will soon be able to see the positive results that are being achieved. There are some blank charts at the back of this book that you can fill in to start your sleep diary.

○   As mentioned in Chapter 3, it is important to put in place a good bath and bedtime routine which gives the signal that sleepy-time is nearly here! Bathtime can often be a lively affair and should always be fun; it is the time after the bath when it is necessary to wind down into a calm, quiet atmosphere. The bedtime routine becomes the focal part of your child's preparation for the night ahead, and even when travelling or away from home if a similar procedure is followed it can still be the trigger for a peaceful night's sleep.

○   It can help to use a baby sleeping bag to keep your baby snug and warm, and to restrict movement slightly, making it harder for an older baby to stand up in his cot.

Taking into account all these guidelines, one of the main factors that contributes to the success of the reassurance sleep-training technique is the removal of all sleep aids or crutches that you and your baby have come to rely on.

A dummy. This is probably the most common sleep aid, but sadly it is often the biggest hindrance to sleep. Many parents find themselves getting up repeatedly throughout the night just to replace the dummy, and I have even seen older babies systematically throw out every dummy put in their cot and then cry in order to ensure a visit from Mum or Dad. If your baby uses a dummy during the day, just at night or even both, then it is best to remove it completely as it is unfair to expect him to learn to sleep without it if he is still allowed to use it for comfort during the day. For a younger baby it is best to take away the dummy at some point during the first day of your sleep-training and any distraction techniques you can think of will need to be used while he re-adjusts to life without it. For an older baby or toddler you can give warning that use of the dummy is going to stop, and make the day you start sleep-training the time that this will happen. It may be that you tell your toddler that tomorrow the 'dummy fairy' is coming and needs to collect all the dummies, or maybe you can let your toddler help to gather up all his dummies and put them into an envelope or a bag that he can decorate and then 'send' to the 'dummy factory' to be recycled. Whatever the age of your baby, there is no doubt that he is going to miss his dummy, but within a matter of days he will forget that it ever existed. Babies up to twelve months will usually have lost the association within two to four days, but older babies and toddlers can take a few days longer.

Mum's the Word . . .

At four and a half months my baby would wake up wanting his dummy and I got into the habit of giving it to him each time he woke, which was three to five times every night! This lasted for about six weeks until I realized I wasn't helping either of us. How could he learn to settle himself when I was doing it for him? I then had to take the dummy away completely, and following Alison's sleep-training method my baby began to sleep for 12 hours within five nights.

J. R.

Dream feed. Following advice from other baby routines, many parents wake their baby in the late evening to offer a dream feed in the hope that this will encourage him to sleep until morning. Although this may seem to work for a few weeks around the three-month stage, I have found that things often regress, with the baby starting to wake more frequently after the feed and earlier in the morning. In fact, I have seen many babies from six to twelve months of age who, though at three months they were sleeping through from the 11pm dream feed to the morning, ended up having another two or three feeds in the night because they expected to be fed every time they woke. By waking your baby for a feed you are giving his body food that he doesn't actually need and causing his digestive system to work overtime, which interferes with his developing sleep habits. So when you decide to start your sleep-training, leave your baby to sleep and do not wake him. Granted, he may wake himself around the time you usually offered the dream feed, or perhaps sometime later on, but when he does it is essential not to give any feed but to carry out the 'sleepy-time' reassurances as explained on pages 171–2.

Night breastfeeds. Many mothers easily fall into the trap of breastfeeding at night for much longer than is necessary as it seems to be a simple solution for comforting their baby back to sleep. Sometimes the night-waking and the baby's demands for the breast will lead the mother to bypass the cot and just take the baby into bed with her for the whole night, even resorting to going to bed as early as 7 or 8pm every evening! As long as your baby is over three months and has had a reasonable weight gain, then there should be no reason for him to need a night feed. It is possible to try reducing the length of time you let your baby feed during the night gradually over a couple of weeks, but to be honest you will find it much easier just to stop all night feeds and replace them with the sleep-training. Yes, your baby may be slightly hungry during the first night or two, and it is emotionally extremely difficult for a mother to stop offering breastfeeds, but if you can summon the resolve to get through that first night or two, the overwhelming urge you may have to keep offering your breast will quickly subside and your baby will soon adapt to not relying on night feeds and learn to take the sustenance he does need during the day.

Night bottlefeeds. As with breastfeeding, many parents can find themselves offering numerous feeds throughout the night in a desperate attempt to re-settle their baby. If you are offering one or more feeds when your baby wakes, it is possible to start watering down the milk you offer in the hope that the baby will become less reliant on food during the night. Whether you are using expressed breast milk or formula, see pages 105 and 112 on how to water down the feeds. However, quicker results will be achieved by going 'cold turkey' and stopping night feeds altogether, replacing them with the reassurance method as explained in this chapter.

Feeding your baby to sleep. Many mothers, especially those who are breastfeeding, have found that their baby will fall asleep while feeding, so they will then transfer him to the cot or to their bed without waking him. When he then wakes throughout the night he will need and expect another feed with which he will settle back to sleep. This can be an easy habit to fall into, but will rarely encourage your baby to sleep for long periods at a time. When you implement the reassurance sleep-training, obviously you will still need to give your baby a feed before he goes to bed, but you will have to ensure that as he goes into his cot he is at least partly awake. Always put him into his sleeping bag after the feed, as this is often enough to wake him sufficiently so that he is aware that he has been moved away from you and put into his cot. If he is extremely sleepy and difficult to rouse after the feed, you may even need to change his nappy to wake him enough. Then you will be able to use the 'sleepy-time' reassurances to settle your baby instead of a breast or bottle.

Drinks of water or juice. Some parents get to the point where they have removed milk feeds during the night only to find they have replaced them by giving their baby numerous bottles or cups filled with water or juice. This tends to happen with older babies or toddlers and sometimes the parents just leave the bottles in the cot for the baby to help himself, assuming that it is not causing too much of a problem. However, in many such cases the child is not getting uninterrupted sleep and this can easily have a negative impact on his daytime behaviour. As with the previous sleep aids mentioned, for the best results it will be necessary to remove these drinks in order to introduce the reassurance sleep-training technique.

Again you may choose to remove these drinks gradually by reducing the liquid volumes and number of bottles or beakers over a few days. After a few nights you should then remove them completely and replace with the sleep training as explained in this chapter.

Music. Many parents will play some soothing music in the nursery while they give their baby the last feed and then leave it playing while the baby settles himself to sleep. Unfortunately this can easily escalate to become a relied-upon sleep aid, as when the baby stirs during the night he needs to hear the same music before he can go back to sleep. Some parents come to rely on music that can be played through their baby-listening monitor, only to find themselves frequently waking throughout the night in readiness to switch on the music as their baby begins to stir. If you wish to have music during the last feed, be sure to turn it off before you put your baby in his cot for the night and replace his dependence on music with your 'sleepy-time' reassurances.

Nightlights. You may feel that it is comforting for your baby to provide some source of low lighting throughout the night. However, I find most babies up to two years of age will actually sleep better in a dark room without any form of nightlight. Some older children may go through a phase of separation anxiety and seem to be comforted by a nightlight, and if they continue to sleep through with this in place then there is little to worry about. If you are using nightlights and your baby is still not sleeping, then it is best to remove them in conjunction with implementing sleep-training.

Mobiles and cot toys. Attractive as these may seem, it is important for your baby to learn that his cot is not a play area but a place to sleep. However, sometimes if you are busy during the day the cot can be a useful place to leave your baby for a few minutes when he is awake and he may be happily entertained by a cot mobile or a few toys, but they must then be removed before putting him down for any nap or nighttime sleep. If he has come to rely on watching a mobile or light show while settling himself to sleep, as with the other sleep aids mentioned you will need to remove it as you start your sleep-training.

Swaddling. In the early weeks swaddling can help a baby feel more secure but, as mentioned in Chapter 3, it is important to remove the swaddle by around six weeks of age. If for any reason you are still using a swaddle for your older baby, it is important to remove it to coincide with the start of sleep-training. You could try gradually loosening the swaddle for a few days leading up to starting the technique so that your baby becomes less reliant on being wrapped so snugly, or you could try putting him on his tummy to sleep as this can help to replace the feeling of security that the swaddle gave. Some parents feel that they have to keep swaddling their baby as he claws and scratches at his face or ears if his hands are free. If this is the case, before you embark on any sleep-training it would be advisable to read Chapters 1 and 3 which explain all about 'sleep behaviour', and also Chapter 7 on reflux/dietary intolerances to ascertain what is causing such behaviour.

Patting, shushing, stroking, holding or rocking. Many parents find that a certain amount of patting, stroking, rocking, etc., is comforting to a young baby and will help to settle him during the early weeks. However, this can easily be overdone and before you know it the only way your baby will drift off to sleep is by being patted, shushed or rocked in your arms. Some other sleep-training methods suggest a gradual withdrawal and advise you to do one fewer pat or rock for one minute less each night and so on, but from my experience a complete withdrawal replaced by my 'sleepy-time' reassurances is far more successful.

Sleeping in the baby's room. An extreme example of some of the above points can result in a parent feeling the need to sleep on the floor or on a mattress next to the baby's cot in order to provide comfort each time he wakes by holding his hand or replacing his dummy. As you start to implement my technique, it will be necessary to stop sleeping in with your baby and replace the comfort you have been giving with the 'sleepy-time' message. As in the previous point, some other methods would suggest a more gradual withdrawal by moving your mattress nearer to the door each night until you are on a chair outside the baby's room, but again I emphasize that a complete 'cold-turkey' withdrawal is much quicker and much more effective when replaced with the 'sleepy-time' reassurances.

Mum's the Word

I gave Jessica her sleep problem – she was born early and I was told to feed her every 2 hours until she reached full-term. During the first night she woke every hour and a half and I fed her and she fell asleep on the breast, therefore she learned from Day 1 that she had to be fed to fall asleep. I was unaware of how much sleep new babies need so wasn't allowing her enough opportunity to sleep. Result, one very tired baby!

Then I realized if I took her for a walk she fell asleep, so I walked with her for 40 minutes every afternoon, but this soon led to me having to walk every time she needed to sleep during the day, which was often up to four hours every day. At night I would settle Jessica in her cot after she had fallen asleep feeding and when she woke I would bring her into my bed to feed her and we would both fall asleep. If I tried to put her back into her cot she would wake and scream, so I didn't bother and she would stay in with me for the rest of the night.

I enlisted Alison's help and she explained how to implement her reassurance sleep-training and from then on we never looked back.

I had been trying to get my baby to sleep in her cot for six months – Alison solved that in just 9 minutes!

I do remember Alison told me that, when I first put Jessica down in her cot and she was screaming, 'she'll still love you afterwards!' And the next morning she greeted me with a huge smile when she woke up and was clearly so proud of herself!

M. Y.

Using a buggy or pram for sleeps. Some parents find that their baby will sleep only in a buggy for any daytime naps and they will have to walk for 3–4 hours each day to ensure he gets enough sleep – good exercise at times, but not when you have to go out no matter what the weather! I have also known a few desperate parents who have resorted to pushing a buggy around the house to get their baby off to sleep but then have to resume pushing throughout the night when he wakes up. Whether you are using the buggy for daytime naps or during the night, from the day you begin implementing the sleep-training it will be necessary to remove the buggy and simply put your baby into his cot and follow the 'sleepy-time' reassurance technique.

Baby sleeping in the parent's bed. During the early weeks you may have decided to bed-share with your baby, or resorted to allowing him to sleep in your bed just to get a few hours' sleep, but now find that you cannot get him to sleep alone in his cot. This is one of the most common scenarios that I come across and it is often the cause of upsets and arguments between partners. It can easily result in parents sleeping in separate bedrooms and feeling that they have lost the intimate part of the relationship they once had. If your baby has never slept in his cot or in his own room, it is a good idea to introduce him to them in the days prior to starting your sleep-training. This can be done by allowing him to have some play time during the day in the room and even in the cot (see page 166), and maybe using his room for nappy changes and as part of his bedtime routine by reading stories in there. The day you start to implement sleep-training you will need to put your baby into his cot for his daytime naps as well as at bedtime and use the 'sleepy-time' reassurances.

Muslin or comforter. Some babies do like to have something to hold and snuggle up with as they sleep and the easiest thing to give them is a muslin square. As muslins are 100 per cent cotton and completely breathable, they are safe for your baby to have with him in his cot where they are easy for him to find. The muslin can become as much a signal to sleep as your 'sleepy-time' message and when you are out and about during a nap time you can recline the pushchair, give your baby his muslin, tell him it is 'sleepy-time' and hopefully he will drift off to sleep.

Now you have reached the point where you are going to put the reassurance sleep-training technique into practice, but before you start do go through the following checklist once more:

○ Your baby is free from illness.

○ He is eating well and has had a sustained weight gain.

○ Any reflux or dietary issues have been diagnosed, treated and managed.

○ You have implemented a good daytime and bath/bedtime routine.

○ He has grown familiar with his room and cot.

○ Dummies have been collected and put away.

○ Toys and mobiles have been removed from the cot.

○ You have a clear diary for the next few days.

○ There is support and understanding from other family members who are closely involved.

○ And just to keep you sane – some earplugs, a bottle of wine and some comfort food to help you through the night! Only joking, but it will help if you can try to keep a sense of humour!

○ You have been keeping a sleep diary for the last few days.

If all the above have been put in place and you feel ready – well, actually, no parent ever feels 'ready' – then the following tells you 'how to do it'.

Implementing the reassurance sleep-training technique

The same 'sleepy-time' messages used in this technique need to be followed for both daytime naps and nighttime sleeping with just a few adjustments for day or night. It doesn't matter whether you start in the morning and sleep-train for the naps during the day first, before carrying it on for bedtime and throughout the night, or if you start at bedtime and sleep-train throughout the night first and then continue for the naps throughout the following day. You will, however, need to read both the following sections, whichever time you choose to start your sleep-training, as you do need to use the technique for both daytime naps and throughout the night from the beginning.

Starting at bedtime

Carry out your bathtime routine as normal and give your baby his last feed. Ideally, this feed should be given in the baby's room in a calm, quiet atmosphere. I fully appreciate that if you have other children to tend to this may prove difficult, but this is why I earlier mentioned about asking for as much help and support from others as possible. It will be useful to have someone else to look after the other children so that you are able to focus on your baby and the task in hand.

In these first few days it may be that it takes up to an hour or so to feed and get your baby settled, but very soon bedtime will become a breeze and he will go straight down and be asleep within minutes, therefore leaving you with time to be with your other children.

After bathtime and before settling down for the feed, close the curtains and lower the lighting if possible. Then directly after feeding your baby and ensuring he has brought up any wind, put him into his sleeping bag and place him in his cot. Turn off any music and the lights, and say to your baby, 'Good night Baby [use his/her name], it's SLEEPY-TIME now,' while maybe stroking or patting him.

The phrase you devise and use is up to you, but it must consist of the same words every time you say it to your baby throughout the sleep-training process and beyond. However, do keep it quite short and to the point, and ensure that anyone else involved in helping you says the same thing. In multilingual families it is best if the phrase is said in the mother's language first and then repeated in the second language during each reassurance visit to settle your baby. My favourite phrase incorporates 'it's sleepy-time' as I find this becomes the focal part of what I say that doesn't change. For example, at bedtime when first putting a baby into his cot I will say, 'Night night, Rory, it's sleepy-time now. Night night.' Then every time I enter the room to re-settle him I will say, 'That's enough now, Rory. It's sleepy-time. Night night.'

When saying goodnight to your baby and putting him into his cot, you might repeat your chosen phrase a few times, making sure your voice is calm, confident and reassuring. When you then have to go back in to reassure him, you need to add the words, 'That's enough now. It's sleepy-time,' saying it in a much firmer tone of voice to convey that you are in control, mean business and are no longer a soft touch. It can be hard to believe, but your baby will respond and react more positively if you sound firm and in control rather than if you try to whisper softly to him in a meek and mild voice. A soft, hesitant tone can instigate feelings of insecurity and uncertainty in your baby, whereas he will be comforted and reassured by Mummy sounding confident, firm and in control, even though you may not feel that you are!

Whatever sleep aid your baby has been used to settling with will now have been removed and you will put him into his cot, say your goodnight phrase, leave the room and close the door behind you. More than likely your baby will start to cry and may even be at full pitch before you can get through the door, but summon all your resolve, ignore him, carry on out of the door and close it behind you.

Alison says . . .

Remember, I did say there might be tears – yours as well as his!

Now, just wait a few minutes and if he doesn't calm down you will need to go in and give a 'sleepy-time' reassurance. Go back into the room, walk over to the cot, place a firm, reassuring hand on him and say your phrase in a strong, firm voice: 'That's enough now. It's sleepy time. Night night,' then immediately leave the room again, closing the door. He may still be crying and may continue to do so for some time, but all you need to do from now on is repeat the 'sleepy-time' reassurance in the same way. Eventually he *will* go to sleep and you can breathe a sigh of relief and may feel like reaching for the champagne! But it is a little early to celebrate, as it's highly likely that your baby will wake again during the night and you will need to repeat the 'sleepy-time' reassurance process. Every time he does wake and you feel that he is not going to re-settle by himself, try to stay calm (anxious as you may feel) and carry on going in and out of his room to reinforce the 'sleepy-time' message. The section on page 181, 'Typical responses to the Reassurance Sleep-training Technique', should help to give you an idea of how often this may happen during the first few nights.

Questions frequently asked about using the reassurance sleep-training technique

Q   *How many minutes should I leave it before going in each time?*

A   This technique is not really about clock-watching or timing the minutes in between each visit to your baby's room. It is more to do with listening to your baby and going in when you feel he really needs a reassurance but leaving him to it when he doesn't. If you always go in and give a reassurance at set intervals of, say, every 4 minutes, your baby will quickly learn the pattern, expect you to appear after that set time and fail to settle to sleep as he will be anticipating your visit. Throughout sleep-training, try to vary the length of time between your visits, sometimes carrying out three reassurances in quick succession and at other times leaving a longer interval.

It's almost as though you need to keep your baby 'guessing' when you will next appear. What does then become clear to him very quickly is that you *will* come and reassure him with the same repeated 'sleepy-time' message, thereby removing his previous confusion and reinforcing one simple message: 'It's sleepy-time.'

Q   *If I am not guided by timed intervals, then when should I go into his room?*

A   As in the previous answer, there is no set pattern or prescriptive routine for when you should go into your baby's room when he is crying. In truth, a lot will depend on his cry and your learning to interpret whether it is of anger, frustration, overtiredness, discomfort or real distress. You may feel that you will never understand what his cry means, but trust your instincts (yes, you *do* have them!) and you will quickly begin to understand what he is saying. There is a difference in every baby's cry, whether he is just having a whinge and a moan, 'shouting' with frustration, 'bellowing' with anger or really crying through discomfort. The fact is that no baby likes change and when you start this sleep-training process he will be confused, upset and possibly angry, which will make him cry, but it is usually very shortlived because he will soon forget his previous associations and learn the new ones you are putting in place. Also be aware that you should resist the urge to go in every time his cry reaches a certain pitch; if you do so he will quickly learn that he needs to reach a particular level of cry to gain your attention.

Try to think of your baby's cry on a scale of one to ten. For some guidance on this, I have devised the following table to help you:

The crying scale	
1	A little whimper: he may grunt and groan on and off for some time, but will not need any reassurance.
2	A small moan: he may whinge and moan a little but will rarely need a visit at this level.
3	An annoyed squawk: he may be getting a little more vocal at this point and just slightly crying, but it is still best to leave him to see if the cry develops or subsides.
4	A frustrated squeal: he may be crying on and off for a few minutes, but with no real conviction and you can actually tell that it is fairly half-hearted.
5	A demanding shout: he may well be loudly vocalizing his displeasure at the turn of events and be missing his dummy, for instance, but the cry is not entirely continuous.
6	An escalating cry: he may now be working up to the point where he will not re-settle himself and you will judge whether it is appropriate to go in and give a reassurance.
7	A panicky distress call: your baby may sound quite distressed and be crying with only a few brief pauses for breath. If you have not been in for a while, now would be a good time to do so.
8	A very angry yell: a baby can sustain crying at this level for some time, but it is usually out of frustration and anger that things have changed and he

doesn't understand why. If you carry out repeated 'sleepy-time' reassurances he will begin to calm down.

---

9   A full-blown cry: if a true full-on cry does not subside after several minutes, you may need to try another tactic and do a quick reassuring 'pick-up and then put-down' along with delivering the 'sleepy-time' message.

---

10   A blood-curdling scream: using my technique no baby ever reaches this point as he has already been reassured. I use number 10 merely to emphasize this scale!

Alison says . . .

After explaining the 'crying scale' to parents, I will then ask them to assess at various times what level of cry they think their baby is at as we start the sleep-training process. Very often what I would put down as a cry at level 3 they will be sure is at least a 5 or 6. This is very common, as crying always sounds so much worse than it actually is – especially to the parents.

Q   *Will my baby 'hate' me for doing this and will it emotionally or mentally scar him?*

A   Nearly every parent asks me this. They have very real fears and anxieties that their baby will be damaged in some way by being put through the changes necessary to undergo the sleep-training process. In actual fact this is not the case and your baby will come out the other side of the sleep-training happier, better rested and more content. They simply do not remember what happens during the first few days of initiating sleep-training and, although they may go through periods of upset and distress at the change, it is very shortlived and soon forgotten as they move into calm and happy sleep within a week or two. Remember, your baby will forget his earlier habits as quickly as he learns the new ones, which also means that, as the upset of change diminishes very quickly, so does any lasting impression of it. Practically all parents whom I have helped with sleep-training have been utterly amazed that their baby appears to have survived the ordeal completely unscathed and even still smiles at them in the morning. You may be feeling a little ragged around the edges, have been worrying all night and imagine it will take an age for you to get over it, but this is certainly not the case for your baby. He is, and will be, fine!

Mum's the Word . . .

My memory is of us putting Thomas to bed at 7pm [at seventeen weeks old] and listening to him cry on the baby monitor, when you asked me on a scale of 1 to 10 how bad I thought it was. I said 8 to 9 but you, very confidently and reassuringly, said it probably wasn't even a 5 and that gave me the strength to keep going and helped me gain some perspective and understand that a new mother may well not be in a very 'objective' state of mind. All I can say is 'Thank you'!

K. W.

Starting at nap time

Nap times can be harder to establish than the unbroken night sleep and will often take slightly longer to fall into place. Whereas in the evening you have your bedtime routine to use as a signal that sleepy-time is soon to follow, there is no real equivalent that can be used for nap times other than a fairly well structured, albeit flexible, daytime routine. You may find it useful to look at the following chart to understand what your baby's daytime sleep requirements may be so that you can work out what naps he should be having.

Age in months	Number of naps	Nap 1	Length of nap	Nap 2	Length of nap	Nap 3	Length of nap
3–6	3	morning	1–2 hours	midday	2 hours	afternoon	30–60 mins
6–9	2–3	morning	45 mins– 1½ hours	midday	1½–2½ hours	This nap is usually the first that your baby will drop.	20–40 mins
9–12	2	morning	½–1 hour	midday	1¾–2½ hours		
12–18	1–2	Your baby may be ready to drop this nap now.		midday	2–3 hours		
18–24	1			midday	2 hours		

Daytime naps

As you have cleared your diary for the next few days, you should use the cot in your baby's room to establish the daytime naps. This does not mean that you will always need to be at home so that your baby can take his naps in his cot; once established, naps can be of a more flexible nature and your baby will get used to taking them in different surroundings.

To begin your sleep-training during the day, as nap time approaches begin to tell your baby what is about to happen. Even if you think he is too young to understand at, say, four months, he will soon start to associate the words you use – 'Time for your nap soon, Rory' – as a signal that nap time is near. Then take your baby to his room, close the curtains, put him into his sleeping bag and then into the cot. Now is the time to use the phrase, 'It's nap time now, Rory, sleepy-time. Night night,' leave the room and close the door. Your response, if your baby cries, is to leave him for a few minutes to see if he starts to calm down and begin to settle. If he does not, you must then start to use the 'sleepy-time' reassurances as described earlier and continue to use the technique until he goes to sleep.

However, during the day you are much more governed by time, so it may sometimes be necessary to end the nap even though your baby has not actually slept. For instance, let's say your baby is six months old and you are putting him down for his first nap of the day at around 9am. Ideally he should sleep for about 60–90 minutes. However, if after 45 minutes of your going in and out giving your 'sleepy-time' reassurances he is still resisting and refusing to settle to sleep, you might decide that both you and he have had enough and end the nap time. To do this you should leave him for a good few minutes without going in at all and then breeze into his room with a happy, bright voice saying, 'Time to wake up now. Haven't you had a lovely sleep?' Now, you might think I am crazy – and your baby may think you are too – but it is so important to end the nap time in this positive way rather than going into his room as a defeated parent and muttering under your breath, 'OK, you win. I'll just have to get you up then.' Even though your baby may not have slept, it is vital that you keep a positive outlook throughout the training as he will easily pick up on any negative attitude or feelings that you have.

Alison says . . .

This is a battle of wills – and one which you **MUST** win!

If your baby didn't sleep and you end the nap time as I have explained, please don't feel that this is a failure on your part and that the sleep-training is not going to work. It will work, but it is quite common for this to happen during the first few days. Hard as it may seem to find the resolve to continue, please don't give up at this first hurdle. Keep to your routine, put your baby down for his next scheduled nap and try again. After his refusal to sleep at the first nap it would be a good idea to take him for a walk or a drive in the car and hope that he might doze off for a short while, as if he doesn't sleep at all he may get so overtired that he finds it even harder to settle for the next nap. Similarly, if your older baby is having only one sleep a day and after an hour or so still refuses to settle when you put him down for his midday nap, I would suggest that you positively encourage a sleep somewhere, somehow during the afternoon. If your baby has no sleep at all it could easily have the knock-on effect of his having a much more disturbed night as he is so overtired.

Referring to the chart on page 177, you will see that younger babies may be having three naps each day. However, I suggest that you use the baby's cot and carry out actual sleep-training only for the first two naps of the day. The third nap will often be somewhere in the late afternoon and I find that it is better to use neither the cot nor the sleep-training so close to bedtime. I feel that using any sleep-training technique more than twice during the day and then again at night can be a bit overwhelming for both you and your baby.

Many babies will sleep only for 40–50 minutes during the day for naps and this is a very common problem. As explained in Chapters 1 and 3, babies sleep in 40–45-minute cycles. They will often stir then wake after the first 40-minute active-sleep cycle, then struggle to settle back down into the next, much needed, quiet-sleep cycle. Although they may take four or five of these brief naps each day, it can still cause them to become overtired as they never get the quality, rejuvenating rest that comes through having the quiet-sleep cycle. During the sleep-training process, if your baby wakes after 45 minutes at nap time, you then have to decide whether to try to get him to go back to sleep or just to end the nap and get him up. It is very difficult for me to be prescriptive about what you should do, but the following examples might give you some guidance:

○ A four-month-old baby, having woken at 6.30am, is put down for Nap 1 at 8.15am and is asleep by 8.30am, but wakes at 9.10am. In this instance, as it is still nearly 2 hours away from the next feed and I instinctively know that the baby is still really tired, I would use the reassurance sleep-training technique to try to get him to go back to sleep. I would continue for at least 30–40 minutes, and maybe even longer, but as the time heads towards 10am I may decide to end nap time and take him out for a walk. Say then that the baby goes to sleep within 10 minutes for Nap 2 at noon and once more wakes after 40 minutes. Again, I would continue with sleep-training for up to an hour and hope that he would go back to sleep. Usually it really does start to improve very quickly and you will find that for at least one of the naps your baby is sleeping through the 40-minute nightmare and staying asleep for a longer period of time.

○   A nine-month-old baby, having woken at 7am, is put down for his nap at 9am and wakes after 45 minutes. In this case I would probably get him up, as 45 minutes for Nap 1 is fairly typical for a baby of this age. However, if he goes down for Nap 2 and still wakes after 45 minutes, I would then continue to encourage him to go back to sleep using the reassurance sleep-training method for at least an hour, as it is Nap 2 that is really important to get established at this age.

When you are trying to decide whether to end nap time or continue with the sleep-training, do take into consideration what your baby's night sleep has been like, what time he woke in the morning, what happened at the previous nap, whether it is nearly feed time, how tired you feel your baby is, etc. You will never get it right all the time, and you may go into the room to end nap time and discover that he is crying only because he is frustrated and really wants to go back to sleep, or you may continue with the 'sleepy-time' reassurances and then discover that he has a poo! Whatever the scenario, don't be too hard on yourself about the decisions you make; as I have said, sometimes you will get it right and sometimes you will get it wrong, but don't worry – there is always the next nap time to come and bedtime beckoning at the end of the day so you can practise the sleep-training technique once more.

> **Mum's the Word . . .**
>
> ❧ My favourite memory is from my first day with Alison, putting
> the twins to bed for a lunchtime nap. They had never slept in
> their cots during the daytime and I was so apprehensive and
> worried. Staring at the video monitors my heart was racing
> and we watched the clock as the twins wriggled and shouted.
> Within 10 minutes Evie had fallen asleep and Oliver followed
> after 30 minutes – it really wasn't so bad. Although it seemed
> remarkably simple using this technique to reassure them, I
> was convinced I couldn't do it on my own. Now here we are,
> nine months later, with a wonderfully structured day and
> plenty of rest for all of us. ❧
>
> A. H.

Typical responses to the Reassurance Sleep-training Technique

It is, of course, extremely difficult to predict how your baby will respond to sleep-training, but to give you some guidance I have collated the results from 100 babies who have undergone my reassurance technique. The length of time it takes for a baby to settle and the amount of times he may wake are listed below, but are obviously only averages for each age group. Please remember it is only a guide – every individual baby responds in a slightly different way and some will adapt to and accept the changes more easily than others.

3–12 months

Often the younger the baby, the more readily he will adapt to the changes and respond with relative ease to sleep-training. This is because his learned habits are not quite so ingrained, so you can expect him to forget a learned association within two or three days and accept the new routine just as quickly.

A typical four-month-old baby may take 20–40 minutes to settle at the first attempt to put him down either for a nap or at night. He may wake anywhere between one and four times during the night, but usually takes less time to re-settle after each wakeful period. It will usually only take two to four days for a baby in this age range to accept and adapt to this method of sleep-training. Usually Night 1 is the most difficult, with the ensuing nights becoming easier as you go through the process, but often Night 1 can be surprisingly easy and you may then find that Night 2 is slightly more challenging. I have worked with many babies who have responded amazingly quickly and have even slept through on Night 1 or 2 of sleep-training.

I have found this quick response to be the most usual and there are only a very few that put up more resistance and take longer than the three-day average. The worst scenario I have come across to date was a seven-month-old baby boy who had suffered from severe reflux. His reflux had not been diagnosed till four months; it then took a long time for it to be brought under control and for the correct medication and formula to be prescribed and take effect. During these months the baby had been unable to sleep comfortably and his parents had resorted to using a number of sleep aids, including a dummy, swaddling, sleeping next to him and offering night feeds every time he woke. A typical night would consist of constant attention from Mum or Dad, hours of crying and little or no sleep for the whole household – or their neighbours! Having removed all the sleep aids and put him into his cot on his own, that first evening of sleep-training it took 2 hours and 20 minutes before he finally slept. He then woke a further three times during the night and it took over an hour each time to get him to re-settle. Over the next few days things gradually improved, but progress was slow and it was a full ten days before he was actually sleeping through the night and readily taking his daytime naps. This was an extreme case and as yet I have not encountered any other baby in this age group who has taken so long to respond.

12–24 months

By this age babies can prove to be a little more resistant to the sleep-training, as the older the child the more deeply ingrained their learned habits and sleep associations, therefore it takes longer for them to adapt to change. Your baby will also be more mobile and will be able to stand up in his cot, so you will need to put him back down firmly into his sleep position at the same time as you deliver your 'sleepy-time' phrase. Often before you even get to the door he will be standing up again, but you must just continue out, shut the door and revisit as necessary, repeating the process. Sometimes it can be useful not to go into the room at all, but to give the 'sleepy-time' reassurance through the closed door or by speaking through a two-way sound monitor, and intersperse this method of delivery with going in and out.

I have witnessed many babies of this age group via a video camera that I put in their room during the sleep-training process and it is fascinating to see how their reactions change as the training progresses. To start with they may be continually standing up and even shaking the bars of the cot with utter frustration, shouting at the tops of their voices, but after a while they run out of steam and can only manage a sitting position, from which they eventually give in and lie down to sleep.

As babies' vocabulary increases it can be hard to resist getting drawn into a conversation with them, but it is really important that you try not to respond to their chatter and just reinforce the 'sleepy-time' phrase. I once witnessed a twenty-month-old girl who after half an hour of crying from the onset of sleep-training decided to use another tactic to get Mummy's attention. When her mother next went into the room the little girl stopped crying immediately and said, 'Pretty top, Mummy,' while giving her a huge grin! It is so difficult to retain control and say the right words when all you want to do is collapse in fits of laughter and give your baby a cuddle!

As a general guide it can take five to seven days for ages twelve to eighteen months and possibly seven to ten days for ages eighteen to twenty-four months before the baby is ready to give in, accept the changes and adjust to the new sleep-filled routine. An example of how easy sleep-training can be was a sixteen-month-old boy who, although having a regular bathtime routine, still rarely settled to sleep in the evening and would wake constantly throughout the night until he was taken to sleep in his parents' bed. In this case the problem stemmed from the parents being in disagreement over the best way to tackle the problem. They had tried countless methods each and every night, and whereas one parent would try to leave the baby in his cot, the other would be quick to pick him up and sleep with him in the spare bed. After explaining my technique and ensuring that both parents agreed that they would fully commit to it, we started sleep-training. The only other thing that we changed was shutting the door to the baby's room. After putting him into his cot on the first night and closing the door, he complained for all of 10 minutes and then went to sleep. That was all we heard from him till 6.30 the next morning. Both parents were in complete shock at such a good result, but I did warn them to be prepared for some regression during the following nights. However, this did not happen and the baby continued to sleep through the night.

Once you have started sleep-training using my reassurance method you may begin to notice some surprising changes in your baby's behaviour. Because his body is learning to relax and beginning to catch up on the sleep it needs, less adrenaline is released into his system, so he becomes less 'wired' and can seem almost more tired than before. This tiredness is displayed by constant yawning, floppiness, nodding off to sleep at odd moments, seeming very soporific and just 'not on this planet', as opposed to the fractious, tense and agitated behaviour he previously showed. Once your baby starts to respond to the training he will actually crave sleep, becoming a complete 'sleep monster' for a few days while his body re-adjusts and catches up. He will then reach his plateau and start to find his own natural sleep pattern and requirements. For guidance on how much sleep your baby may need, see the tables on pages 72 and 177.

Early-morning waking

There are four main types of early-morning waking in babies. The first may occur during the first few days of the sleep-training process while your baby's sleep patterns are lengthening to the magical 12-hour night sleep. The second is when a baby has been sleeping through the night for some time but suddenly starts to wake early for no apparent reason. The third is that the baby has never slept the full 12 hours and has always woken early, between 5 and 6am. The fourth could be that as a baby gets older he starts to need less sleep during the day, so it may indicate that it is time to drop one of his daytime naps.

Type 1

Having implemented the reassurance sleep-training technique, you may be faced with the situation of your baby waking around 5am. If you have removed any night feeds and this happens on the first night, you may find it extremely difficult to resist offering a feed, but it is best not to do so and to persevere with your 'sleepy-time' reassurances. Your baby will be absolutely fine – waiting another hour or so for his feed will have no detrimental effect on him at all. Whatever other sleep aids have been removed, including the unnecessary night feeds, if your baby wakes any time before 6am then you should just treat it as nighttime waking and continue with your sleep-training. However, if it gets to 6am and beyond, you may have been carrying out your 'sleepy-time' reassurances for some time and it is now obvious that your baby is not going to settle, or quite simply you may have had enough and want to start the day. In this case you need to follow the same pattern for ending a nap time. Leave your baby without visiting his room for a few minutes, then go in using a bright and breezy voice, say 'Good morning' to him, open the curtains and go to the cot to greet him. As with nap time, it is important to use a happy, light voice for this morning greeting as opposed to the firm, confident tones used when delivering the 'sleepy-time' message.

It may be that your baby wakes around 6am and in this case, rather than continuing to deliver the 'sleepy-time' message, it is best to try to leave him for as long as possible before going in to start the day. During the first few nights of sleep-training it is fairly common for a baby to wake early, and after having woken and re-settled at various times throughout the night it is better to start your day a bit earlier rather than continue with the 'sleepy-time' reassurance just in order to reach 7am. During the following days and weeks, as your baby develops his own regular sleep pattern he should soon stretch longer throughout the night without waking until he sleeps until around 7am each morning. Some babies go even longer and become 13-hour-a-night sleepers. If your baby falls into this category, make the most of it – but don't boast about it too much or you may become unpopular with other mums who are still struggling! Of course, you can always refer them to this book!

Type 2

If your baby has been sleeping through the night for some time and has unexpectedly started waking early in the morning, then you need to try to find out why. It may be that he is having a growth spurt and you will need to increase his feeds to match his growth. However, this is usually only shortlived and he will soon revert to his normal waking time. Or it may be that he is waking through hunger and it is time to introduce solids into his diet to help sustain him. This is the most probable cause of early-morning waking for a baby aged between four and six months. It could be that your baby is actually not getting enough sleep during the day and therefore is overtired. It is a very strange phenomenon that if a baby does not get enough daytime sleep it will have a negative impact on his night-time sleep, whereas a baby who sleeps really well during the day will often sleep better at night. If your baby struggles to sleep well during the day, then you will need to carry out the reassurance sleep-training technique to get his required daytime naps established. Once his structured daytime naps are in place, you should see an improvement in his sleep at night and this should then eradicate the early-morning waking.

Type 3

Another cause of early-morning waking can be that your baby is not going to bed early enough in the evening and is therefore overtired and struggling to achieve the 12-hour stretch through the night. This is fairly common where parents try to keep their baby awake in the evening so that the working parent can spend some time with the baby on arriving home.

It is a sad fact of life that due to job commitments a working mum or dad may only be able to spend quality time with their children during weekends or days off. This is a harsh reality of the lives we choose to lead and trying to keep a baby up later in the evening when he really needs to go to bed is a double-edged sword. Even though you might think your baby will benefit from seeing the parent for a short while each evening, if he is overtired because of being kept up then ultimately it will have a detrimental effect on his sleep and therefore on his development and wellbeing. Sleep deprivation is the cause of many problems in growing babies and it would be better to have an earlier bedtime that is beneficial to him rather than being kept awake only to spend a fractious few minutes with the parent coming in from work.

If your baby is waking too early in the morning then do consider bringing his bedtime forward by half an hour or so, even if this means he will actually be in bed by 6.30 or even 6pm. This is usually necessary only for a few months during the first year; as he gets older he will be able to have a slightly later bedtime, between 7 and 8pm, without it impacting on his nighttime sleep.

Putting your baby to bed earlier in the evening may mean that he will wake even earlier in the morning, maybe around 4am. Don't panic if this happens, but resort to implementing the reassurance sleep-training technique and after a few days the problem should be solved.

Type 4

It is very difficult to give you an exact time when your baby needs to drop one of his daytime naps. All babies are complete individuals and whereas one twelve-month-old may still want and need two daytime naps, another at nine months may already have adapted to taking just one nap in the middle of the day. For some general guidance on suggested daytime naps for individual age groups, see the table on page 177.

If your baby is still having more than one nap during the day and has started to be unsettled during the night, causing him to wake earlier than usual, then you will need to take into consideration his age, feeding pattern and the amount of sleep he is getting during the day and decide whether it is time to drop one of the daytime sleeps. If you are unsure about this, but unable to discover any other reason why he is waking too early, then you can lose nothing by at least trying it for a few days. If it solves the problem, then all well and good, but if things seem to go from bad to worse then re-establish the daytime nap and read through the rest of this chapter to try to ascertain the cause and how else to combat it.

Tips, hints and reminders

I have summarized the following tips and hints for quick reference to help guide you through the process of implementing the reassurance sleep-training technique.

Although I have repeated some of the previous points and highlighted some other tricks of my trade, please make sure to read the whole of this chapter and do not just work from these quick tips as they are specifically designed only to help reinforce your understanding of the technique.

- Clear your diary for the first week or so of implementing the technique.
- Remove all relied-upon sleep aids.
- Discuss using the technique with others in your family before starting and ensure everyone involved is in agreement and ready to give support.
- Make sure your baby is fit and well.
- If possible, put your baby in his own room and preferably don't have him sharing with siblings throughout the sleep-training process.
- It is best to use a baby sleeping bag instead of sheets and blankets, as not only do they stay in place and keep the baby snug, but they can restrict movement slightly and make it more difficult for an older baby to stand up in his cot.
- Remember to use a strong, firm and confident voice when delivering the 'sleepy-time' message.
- Don't be tempted to engage in conversation with your toddler while sleep-training, but just stick to saying your 'sleepy-time' message. Some babies will try talking to you as a way to get a response and it can be very hard to ignore their chatter, but stick to your guns and wait until you leave the room to laugh at their cunning attempts to throw you off track!
- Use a light, happy voice for the 'good morning' greeting and when you need to end nap time.
- Keep your reassurance visits brief and controlling.
- Vary the regularity of your reassurance visits.

- Use the same 'sleepy-time' phrase for both night and day sleeps.
- Make sure everyone who is involved with the sleep-training uses the same 'sleepy-time' phrase.
- As the sleep-training progresses, sometimes 'less is best' with regard to going in and out of the room and you should make your visits far less frequent.
- Always close the baby's bedroom door and leave it closed while he is asleep.
- Once your baby has gone to sleep don't be tempted to keep going in just to check on him. This nearly always disturbs babies and may cause them to wake.
- If you have a two-way sound monitor then sometimes, instead of going into the baby's room, you can deliver your 'sleepy-time' message through the talk system.
- The more sleep your baby gets, the more easily he will develop regular sleep patterns.
- Never worry that it is too late in the day for your baby to take a nap while he adjusts to his new routine. If naps have been disastrous one day, then it is better for him to have some sleep rather than none and if he wants to sleep between 4 and 6pm, let him – it will make your bath and bedtime easier to manage.
- It can be very useful to keep a sleep diary for a couple of weeks leading up to the start of sleep-training and then continue it for the actual week or so of training. At the back of this book you will find some blank charts which you can use for your diary. In the first instance it can help you to ascertain where the main problems may be, and then it can give you a big confidence boost as you start to see the positive improvements in your baby's sleep patterns as the training progresses. The following example is of a sleep diary for a six-month-old baby girl who was still being breastfed throughout the night, using a dummy to settle to sleep and often ended up going into bed with Mum in the early hours. The baby was fit and well with a good weight gain, had started on some solid food at five months and was eating well. However, she would often cry throughout the day and night and little would comfort her. During the day she would take only short naps in her pram and would not

sleep if put into her cot. On the first day of sleep-training all the dummies were put away and the sleep-training began at midday for Nap 2. The part of the sleep diary shown here starts on Day 1 of sleep-training.

Sleep	Time	Details	Total sleep time
Tues Nap 2	11.30am	Put in cot, cried on and off for 45 mins, went in about 12 times, then slept for 40 mins. Stirred and cried for 3 mins but didn't go in, slept for an hour.	1 hour 40 mins
Nap 3	3.45pm	Went out walking, slept in pram from 3.45 to 4.40pm.	55 mins
Bedtime	6.45pm	Bath 6pm, feed 6.15pm. Into cot at 6.45pm, cried for 35 mins, went in 6 times, asleep at 7.20pm.	
Woke	12.15am	Cried 50 mins, went in about 10 times, crying level never more than 6 on scale!	
Woke	2.30am	Cried 20 mins, only went in 3 times, as more moaning than crying.	
Woke	5am	Cried 35 mins then slept for another hour.	
Wed Woke	6.35am	Started day at 6.45am and fed at 7am. She was very happy and full of smiles. Can't believe she spent whole night in cot!	9 hours 30 mins

Sleep-training diary

Sleep	Time	Details	Total sleep time
Wed Nap 1	8.15am	She was so tired but still took 40 mins to go off with several visits. Then slept soundly till 11.10am	2 hours 15 mins
Nap 2	12.45pm	Moaned for 10 mins, went off to sleep till 1.40pm, woke and cried for 15 mins, 4 visits and she went back for 30 mins.	1 hour 15 mins
Nap 3	3.30pm	Slept 50 mins in pram from 4pm.	50 mins
Bedtime	6.30pm	Bath 5.45pm and feed 6.05pm. Took 20 mins to go to sleep.	
Woke	3.10am	Protested for 45 mins, very cross! Then went back to sleep till 6.10am!	
Thurs Started day	6.55am	Woke at 6.10 but chatted and dozed on and off till I went in at 6.55am.	11 hours

This baby girl responded to the sleep-training very well and, except for the odd 5 or 10 minutes of crying here and there, she slept through the night and happily went into her cot for her daytime sleeps.

This is a fairly typical example of how a six-month-old baby will relatively easily forget the old learned sleep associations and accept the new.

Troubleshooting and avoiding pitfalls

The bedtime feed

If your baby does not take much of his bedtime feed, you may find it difficult to carry out sleep-training because you feel that he may be hungry throughout the night. If this happens and he doesn't settle straight away or dozes for a short time and then wakes up crying, you can re-offer the feed just once to see if he will take any more. It is best to set a time limit of, say, an hour after going to bed to re-offer the bedtime feed. If your baby does take some feed, then as soon as he has finished put him back to bed and continue with the sleep-training. If, however, he refuses the feed, do not be tempted to keep trying to get him to take it. Just put him back to bed and carry on with your 'sleepy-time' reassurances. If you do feel concerned that he is hungry, it might help you to re-read the section on removing nighttime feeds (see pages 105 to 112).

Nap times

These can often take longer to become established than the nighttime sleep. However, it is important that you persevere with the sleep-training and do not give up because if your baby continues not to get enough daytime sleep it may eventually have a negative impact on his nighttime sleep and he may start waking during the night once more.

The crying trap

This is an easy pitfall that can be hard to avoid. As you open the door to go into your baby's room to deliver a 'sleepy-time' reassurance, he may stop crying straight away, only to start again as soon as you turn away to walk out. It is very tempting to turn back to reassure and comfort him again and stay with him for longer periods because you know that as soon as you turn away he is going to cry. Although it may be very difficult to ignore the cry and continue with your controlled, brief visits in and out of the room, it is really important to summon your resolve and stick to using the technique. If you allow your baby to use his cry as a method of drawing you in, it will end up with your baby dictating his own terms and being in control instead of you!

Wind

Many parents worry that after they have put their baby down he starts crying because he has wind and is in discomfort. Usually you can tell if this is the case, either through a difference in the cry or because you know that he did not bring up much wind after the last feed. If you have put your baby to bed, whether it is for a nap or at bedtime, and you feel that he does need to bring up some wind, then as you go in to deliver a 'sleepy-time' reassurance pick him up and wind him but without any further conversation except repeating the 'sleepy-time' phrase as you put him back down.

Dribble

Some babies do produce a lot of saliva, especially when teething, and a mixture of dribble and tears can make the sheet quite damp. If you are using a sleeping bag as I advise, the easiest thing to do when you go in to deliver a 'sleepy-time' reassurance is to move your baby to a dry part of the bottom sheet. As you are not using a top sheet and blankets, the 'feet to foot' position (i.e. putting the baby's feet at the foot of the cot, to stop him wriggling down under the covers) is not relevant.

Vomit

If your baby is sick in his cot and you need to change his bedding, try to do so with the minimum of disturbance and without too much interaction with him. Some babies are prone to be a bit sick or to posset a lot, but a small amount of sick can easily be wiped up as you enter to give a 'sleepy-time' reassurance. A few babies, after crying for even just a few minutes, can almost 'vomit to order'. You will need to clear up, change the bedding and clothing only as necessary, put your baby back into his cot as quickly as possible without offering any further feed and continue with your sleep-training.

Of course, if your baby has been sick and appears to be unwell, you will need to adapt accordingly. For more guidance, see 'Illness and teething' below.

Nappy changing

If at any time you think your baby has done a poo and needs a clean nappy, make the change quickly and calmly, put him back into his cot as soon as possible and continue with your sleepy-time training. You may need to use a larger-size nappy as your baby starts to sleep through the night because obviously he will be going for a longer period of time without being changed. If you find he is being disturbed by wetting through his nappy, you can try putting on a second, larger nappy over the first. Some older babies can almost force themselves to have a poo to ensure that they get your attention, but don't be alarmed by this behaviour – it is quite common, and you just need to change his nappy as quickly and as calmly as possible and put him straight back to bed. I have seen many babies try this tactic and tell you they have had a poo even when they haven't! Don't allow yourself to be 'drawn in': just check his nappy as necessary, using only your 'sleepy-time' reassurances rather than any other conversation.

Illness and teething

As previously mentioned, you do need to make sure your baby is fit and well before instigating sleep-training. Once he is sleeping through the night and readily taking his daytime naps, if he gets ill or is disturbed by the onset of teething it may cause him to wake during the night. While trying to comfort their unhappy baby, parents can easily fall into the trap of offering a night feed, some other sleep aid or taking him into bed with them while he is ill. Of course these are natural reactions, as you will do anything to try to make your baby feel better, but this can easily lead to him then expecting a night feed or wanting to sleep in with you once he has recovered.

If your baby does become unwell and needs extra attention during the night, it is best not to take him out of his room but to sit and comfort him, give him any medicine he needs or maybe a drink of water, all while staying in the nursery. You may even want to put a comfy chair in the room or some cushions on the floor as a place for you to sit with your baby during the time that he is ill, but, as often as you can, keep trying to re-settle him in his cot. As any pain relief medicine you may have given him takes effect, it should help to settle him down fairly easily.

If your baby becomes ill during the first few days of using the technique, you will have to make a judgement on whether to continue your sleep-training or temporarily suspend it until he is better. It should not be necessary to re-introduce any of the night feeds or sleep aids that were originally removed, but just follow the guidelines set out above.

Travelling

Once your baby is regularly sleeping through, it is usually fairly easy for him to adapt to a change of routine and environment when you go away. However, where possible stick to his usual daytime sequence of feed and nap times, and use your 'sleepy-time' message for naps and nighttime as these will reassure your baby and give him the signal to sleep. If you are travelling abroad and need to adjust to different time zones, it is usually relatively easy for your baby to adapt on the outward journey but it can be harder to get back to normal time on your return. When planning your trip try to ensure that you have a few spare days after your return so that you and your baby can re-adjust. You may have to resort to using the reassurance sleep-training technique to get him back to normal.

The same rule applies for babies as for adults when adjusting to different time zones: try to adapt to the local time of your destination as quickly as possible, starting as soon as you get on the plane. It may mean that that you really have to stretch out the day with an extra milk or solid feed and slot in an extra nap, carrying out a bath and bedtime routine to coincide with local time. If you travel overnight but still arrive in the evening local time, it may be best to wake your baby and give extra feeds while you are on the plane so that you can then do bath and bedtime when you arrive. Whatever your travel itinerary, if you have followed my Sensational Baby Sleep Plan from the early weeks and your baby has learned and responds to the key signals for feed time, naps, bath and bedtime, then it will be much easier for you to help him adjust his body clock than if he had no established routine in the first place.

Hour change

Just as everything seems to fall into place and your baby is settled in his routine and sleeping through, around comes that time of year when we have to change the clocks. When this occurs – as with adjusting to time zones – it shouldn't be too difficult for your baby to adapt, especially if he is already in a good routine. There are two ways to deal with the hour change: firstly by 'soaking up' the time difference during the day that it occurs by starting your day as near to the adjusted time as possible, and secondly by adjusting the timing of each day gradually (a couple of days before the hour change and a couple after) by around 15 minutes so that you end up on the new time schedule. If your baby struggles to adjust and continues to wake early then just implement the sleep-training technique as explained in this chapter, paying particular attention to the section on early-morning waking.

Do remember that, although there are some strict rules you must stick to when using this reassurance sleep-training method, all babies are individuals and will respond in slightly different ways. You will need to adapt the technique accordingly and as you progress with the sleep-training you will begin to discover what prompts a positive response from your baby and what doesn't. For instance, after the initial upset at the start of sleep-training, some babies will be reassured by the visits in and out of their room and will settle quickly, whereas others may seem to get more upset and agitated by the frequent interruptions and will respond more positively to the 'sleepy-time' messages being delivered through a two-way monitor or from outside their closed bedroom door.

All that remains is for me to wish you the best of luck and for you and your baby to enjoy all the peaceful, sleep-filled nights that will come once you have got through the whole sleep-training process.

☆ *Alison's Golden Rules* ☆

1   Ensure that your baby is well and not suffering from any degree of digestive discomfort before implementing sleep-training.

2   Make sure you have a good feeding pattern in place during the day and your baby is getting enough milk/food to sustain him through the night.

3   You will need to use this reassurance technique for both the structured daytime naps and throughout the night.

4   Remove all sleep aids or 'crutches' that your baby has come to rely upon and associates with sleep, replacing them with your 'sleepy-time' reassurances.

5   Devise your 'sleepy-time' phrase and always use it throughout sleep-training and beyond. Also make sure that other people involved with your baby's sleep times use the same phrase.

6   Try to enlist some help and support from your husband, partner or other close family members.

7   Ensure that everyone involved with the care of your baby understands the technique and how to use it for both daytime and nighttime sleeps.

8   Clear your diary for the following week or so when you begin sleep-training.

9   Persevere and try not to give in by reverting to previous techniques of getting your baby to sleep.

10   Have faith, steel yourself and go for it! You will be surprised at how easily your baby will respond and you will then reap the benefits of long, sleep-filled nights for years to come.

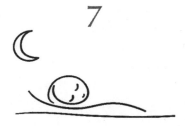

Gastro-oesophageal Reflux and Dietary-related Intolerances

During the early years of my work as a maternity nurse, I soon came to realize that there is a condition in babies that is little understood, often misdiagnosed, sometimes not diagnosed at all, dismissed as an extreme-anxiety condition in an 'overly neurotic mother', ignored by some health professionals because 'babies will grow out of it' and often not even accepted or treated as a medical condition at all. However, for many parents the effects of coping with a baby with this condition, if it is left untreated, can be absolutely devastating.

Instinctively many parents feel that there is 'something wrong' or 'not quite right' with their baby, but after being repeatedly dismissed by their local health professionals they find themselves left with nowhere to turn. Many will research information on the internet, read books or just ask other mums for their opinions but, because every baby will display different signs and symptoms, it can sometimes be almost impossible for the untrained eye to pinpoint what the problem actually is. This is also why many health professionals can find it equally hard to diagnose it in individual babies.

Throughout the last few years I have been trying to raise awareness of this condition among parents and health professionals alike and hope that this chapter will give some much needed understanding, advice and guidance on how to spot, diagnose, manage and treat the condition of gastro-oesophageal reflux and any dietary-related intolerances in babies.

Often these babies are labelled as:

○ sicky
○ screamers
○ difficult
○ colicky
○ challenging
○ poor sleepers

Many people raise the questions of why reflux seems to be becoming such a problem these days and does it truly exist as a medical condition? Some even label it as just a 'trendy' thing for babies to have. My answers are quite simple:

○ Infants have always had reflux, but for many years it was little understood and not really recognized as a medical condition in babies. Thank goodness the majority of the medical world has changed its thinking on the subject during the last twenty years.

○ Due to more people being aware that reflux does exist as a condition in babies, it is becoming a more common topic for discussion within parenting networks.

○ Years ago, most babies slept either on their side or their front, which was a much more comfortable sleep position for those suffering with reflux. Nowadays, since the Back-to-Sleep Campaign launched in the mid-1990s to try to help reduce the incidents of cot death, the advice is to sleep babies only on their backs (see Chapters 1, 3, 4 and 5 for my views on sleep position). This is unfortunately a very uncomfortable position for most babies with reflux, and as a result many do not sleep well or even at all. This can result in them becoming extremely overtired, which undoubtedly has a huge negative impact on the severity of their reflux symptoms . . . not forgetting that the parents are suffering from total sleep deprivation too (see Chapters 1, 3 and 5 for more information on the effects of sleep deprivation).

The colic myth explained

Interestingly, there is much written about so-called 'colic' in babies and everyone seems to have an opinion on it. I have found that many babies are diagnosed as having colic, but this can mean very little in reality as there is no medical definition for the term and it is really just a non-descriptive word for pain. For example, the *Oxford English Dictionary* states:

> **colic** *n*. A severe, spasmodic abdominal pain.

Colic is usually defined as 'excessive crying in infancy with no known cause', but I believe there is nearly always a reason for bouts of inconsolable and excessive crying. The key is to determine the cause and treat accordingly. When diagnosing colic, doctors will often use the 'rule of threes' to decide whether crying is excessive: 3 hours of crying, three or more times a week and having started at around Week 3, with their prognosis then being that there is no need to worry as the baby will grow out of it at around three months of age. This 'rule of threes' is really not particularly helpful: any excessive crying in young babies should be taken more seriously and thoroughly investigated.

Some researchers who studied crying babies diagnosed with colic believe that many of them were actually suffering from reflux and/or digestive intolerances or allergies.

I feel that if 'colic' is still to be used as a term to describe a condition in babies, then it should be re-defined and given a more specific label rather than being used as just an umbrella term for any digestive discomfort. At least by putting some definition for the term in place it would give parents and health professionals some concrete understanding of the likely cause if the baby appears to be 'colicky'. They would then be able to follow a clearer path of management and treatment to help relieve the symptoms.

Further to this, in my experience most babies who appear to be suffering some degree of digestive discomfort and have been labelled as having colic are actually often suffering with either cow's-milk protein and/or lactose intolerance. This, in turn, exacerbates the condition known as gastro-oesophageal reflux. In fact, colic is referred to only twice in the manual *Breastfeeding: a Guide for Midwives* by Dora Henschel and Sally Inch, once with regard to 'cow's-milk protein allergies and intolerances' and once with regard to 'excess lactose', both of which cause 'colic-like' symptoms.

At present colic is sometimes defined as uncontrollable, extended crying in babies who are otherwise healthy and well fed. All babies do cry, as we have seen, but when they cry for more than 3 hours a day, three to four days a week, they are said to have colic. However, it is extremely important to rule out reflux as a cause of this crying, as it is becoming widely acknowledged that many cases of 'colic' are actually undiagnosed and untreated cases of reflux. In these cases, simply treating the reflux may often then eliminate the colicky symptoms that were being displayed.

However, others suggest that the crying is linked to a combination of the baby's temperament and an immature nervous system. They say that the baby's temperament may make him highly sensitive to his environment and it may take him longer to adjust to his surroundings and therefore he reacts by crying, often for long periods. Others believe that endless crying can be linked to the baby having had a traumatic birth experience and it may take up to three months for him to recover. There is very little research or evidence that actually links any of the above to a baby's crying, which in my experience can nearly always be traced to some degree of reflux, 'silent reflux' (see pages 214–17) and/or dietary-related intolerances as opposed to these other explanations.

The problem for parents who are told that their baby has colic is that, because it is not defined as a medical problem, there is no real solution or treatment and they are no better off than they were before seeking help. A variety of self-help tips may be suggested, but on the whole they are told 'not to worry as your baby will grow out of it'. For those who then still face trying to cope with a baby who cries inconsolably for any length of time and rarely settles to sleep, this can be a devastating prospect. The emotional stress, sleep deprivation, inability to help and calm their crying baby, often coupled with feeding problems, have the potential to become the most stressful, unmanageable, self-doubting, isolating, extremely anxious, highly emotional and immensely pressurized situation that they have ever faced. Knowing that the time spent with their new baby is supposed to be the happiest and most fulfilling of their lives will often only add to the emotional turmoil in which the parents already find themselves and it can leave them feeling more confused and stressed than ever. Certainly not the idyll that we often imagine the first steps into parenthood to be!

Living with reflux

The first thing to understand about reflux is that it is rarely 'cured' as a condition and the symptoms it causes truly disappear only as the baby's system develops enough to outgrow them. It is possible to treat, manage and curtail the symptoms through a specific path of treatment and feeding techniques, but these must be monitored under expert advice. Living with reflux is a complete rollercoaster ride for both babies and parents, and often, just as things seem to settle down and a period of relative calm ensues, the symptoms suddenly seem to reappear with a vengeance and everything goes haywire again.

For parents trying to cope with a baby who continually screams, vomits, either doesn't eat or feeds continually, or doesn't sleep, the 'helpful' tips they are often given actually have the opposite effect and send them into the depths of despair:

○ 'Don't worry, all babies cry!'
○ 'It's probably just colic and it gets better at three months.'
○ 'It's OK – they all grow out of it in the end.'
○ 'Just leave him to cry it out. He'll soon get the message!'
○ 'There can't be much wrong, he looks so healthy.'
○ 'Oh, he's just being a bit naughty. You need to put him in a strict routine.'
○ 'Well, his weight gain is OK, so there's no need to worry really.'
○ 'I know he hasn't gained much weight, but some babies are just made to be small.'
○ 'If he doesn't want his feed, why worry? He's obviously not hungry.'
○ 'Maybe it's because you gave up breastfeeding?'
○ 'Reflux? It doesn't really exist, does it?'

As more health professionals are made aware of reflux and begin to understand and then accept it as a serious condition, it is to be hoped that help and support for parents and diagnosis and treatment for babies will soon become more readily available.

◖ Mum's the Word . . .

We had been pushed from pillar to post with our screaming baby and felt like total amateurs – and also as if we were putting people out with our incessant questions. It felt as if we were not taken seriously as there was no way we could have possibly known what is or isn't normal for a very young baby. How wrong they were. WE knew perfectly well that our little boy had a lovely disposition and that the screaming was not with wind, colic or our imagination, but that something was seriously wrong.

When we called Alison we were on our knees, but after taking advice from her (even though she was on holiday!) we followed up her suspicions and managed to find a doctor who understood and confirmed that our little baby had severe reflux and milk intolerances. We continued to take advice and help from Alison and she also helped us to then get our baby to sleep through the night.

Without her help, advice and support I dread to think where we would all have ended up!

A. O.

Reflux explained

The full name for this condition is gastro-oesophageal reflux, or GOR, and the more serious condition is gastro-oesophageal reflux disease, or GORD (these are known as GER and GERD, respectively, in the USA, where they spell oesophagus without the 'o'). The term 'reflux', which means 'backward flow', is a shorter way of referring to GOR and literally refers to the backward flow of stomach contents up into the oesophagus. It is a physiological process that occasionally occurs in everyone, young and old alike, although not everyone is aware of it happening to them.

The oesophagus is basically a long tube that transports food and liquid from the mouth down into the stomach, where at the lower end it connects to the stomach via a valve called the lower oesophageal sphincter, or LOS. This sphincter opens when you swallow to let the foods and liquids pass through and should then close to keep the stomach contents inside. When the LOS doesn't function properly – and in babies this is often simply because of a developmental immaturity – it allows the stomach contents to flow back into the oesophagus to varying degrees. The reflux material may just flow into the lower end of the oesophagus (the distal), move further up towards the throat and sometimes enter the mouth and be ejected as vomit. Most babies do spit up or vomit a little at times, but this rarely causes a problem and will not usually require any medical intervention.

GORD is a more serious complication of the same reflux issue and is often referred to as acid reflux, which is the cause of heartburn. This is when the reflux material not only consists of the stomach contents but also has a high level of hydrochloric acid. This acid is naturally produced in the stomach to aid the digestion of food, but whereas the stomach has a protective lining that acts as a barrier to the acid, the oesophagus, throat, nasal passages, lungs and teeth do not and, over time, repeated exposure to the acid can cause severe pain, increasing damage and some more serious complications.

The majority of babies are born with some degree of reflux simply from the immaturity of the LOS. Although many of them will not experience any pain or heartburn and will outgrow it within a year without the need for medical intervention, many others do suffer with severe symptoms, experience discomfort and pain and will need a definite diagnosis, an ongoing management plan of the condition and appropriate medical treatment.

In the rest of this chapter, as in previous sections of the book, I use the simple term 'reflux' to describe the condition and complications of GORD and acid reflux. Although GORD is a serious condition which needs medical intervention, personally I do not find that labelling reflux with the word 'disease' is very helpful, as many parents then imagine that the problem is far more sinister and also that it is something they have done which has caused their baby to suffer with or to have caught it. If you look at the definition of 'disease' in the *Oxford English Dictionary*, it states:

> **disease** *n*. An unhealthy condition of the body, plant, or some part thereof, caused by infection, diet, or the *faulty functioning of a physiological process* [my italics].

I have actually found that few people understand 'disease' to mean 'a faulty functioning of a physiological process' (which is what GORD is), but just believe it to mean 'an unhealthy condition caused by infection' or something that you 'catch'. The term can then induce much confusion in relation to GORD.

Reflux itself is a simple physiological process, as I have explained, but for many babies who suffer more severe symptoms the following factors also need to be taken into consideration as they can have an impact on the individual baby's symptoms:

- sleep position
- feeding position
- lack of basic daily feeding and sleeping pattern
- overtiredness/sleep deprivation
- stressed atmosphere
- lack of diagnosis
- breast milk
- formula
- lactose intolerance
- cow's-milk protein intolerance
- cow's-milk protein allergy

Reflux often becomes quite a complex problem that can then take patience, understanding, help and support, along with some expert knowledge and often medical intervention, to resolve for each individual baby displaying the signs and symptoms.

Alison says . . .

I always say that you have to 'crack the reflux code' for each individual reflux baby.

Signs and symptoms of reflux

There are many signs of reflux and every baby will display slightly different symptoms according to his condition and its severity. In addition, the behaviour he displays in response to his reflux can be governed by his temperament and individual personality. For instance, some babies cry, some don't; some babies eat well, some don't; some babies sleep well, some don't; some babies still smile, some don't, etc.

The following is a list of the most common symptoms and their usual cause:

- Bouts of inconsolable crying: usually due to the baby being in pain from acid burning, but often exacerbated by being unable to sleep, resulting in extreme overtiredness.
- Appearing to be in pain and distress with little that will comfort him: usually due to the heartburn caused by the reflux of stomach acid.
- Moans and complains most of the time and is rarely happy: often due to feeling wretched because of his constant discomfort.
- Irritable, agitated, rarely relaxed and appears 'wired' a lot of the time: due to the release of extra adrenaline which the body produces to try to deal with the continual pain.
- Body temperature may be slightly higher than normal and the baby may often appear quite hot and clammy: due to the increased adrenaline produced by the body in response to pain.
- Frequent hiccups which sometimes appear to be painful: caused by the spasm of the diaphragm in reaction to the reflux of stomach acid. The baby may also have had frequent and violent hiccups while in the womb, which can be a very early indication that he will suffer from acid reflux.
- Very hard to wind and does not easily burp: because the baby learns very quickly that anything that comes up hurts. He therefore becomes 'retentive' with his wind and rarely burps.
- Continual wet burps or constant spitting up even an hour or so after a feed: due to the slow digestion of the stomach contents and the poor function of the immature LOS.
- Arching the back and neck as if trying to pull away from his chest: due to pain caused by the heartburn.
- Body goes rigid and stiff, it always seems as though the baby is trying to stand up on you, and he becomes muscularly quite strong at a very young age: due to constantly tensing and flexing his muscles through suffering continual pain and discomfort.
- Displaying stress-related behaviour as a reaction to pain or discomfort, such as head-thrashing (as if saying 'No!'); violently rubbing together heels and/or feet, often making the ankles and surrounding skin extremely red and sore; clawing at his head, ears and face, often leaving nasty scratch marks; tugging at his hair and

even pulling it out; violently thrashing his legs up and down or flailing his arms around.

○ Small amounts of vomit produced all the time: caused as the stomach contracts to digest the feed and small amounts are pushed back up into the oesophagus and mouth as the weak LOS fails to remain closed and contain the stomach contents.

○ Projectile vomiting at least once a day: again due to a very weak and immature LOS.

○ Is never sick but displays other symptoms which can indicate 'silent reflux': see pages 214–17.

○ Agitated and fussy over feeds and never seems to relax when feeding: may be due to having a sore oesophagus and/or throat caused by the excess acid.

○ Continually pulling off the breast or bottle: although the baby wants to feed, he quickly associates feeding with discomfort.

○ Head bobbing, like a woodpecker, when put to the breast: again possibly due to the baby already associating pain with feeding.

○ Voraciously suckles for a short while, appearing to be almost 'greedy'; may also be really noisy while feeding, appearing to gulp and guzzle the milk rather than drinking in a calm, relaxed manner: could be due to the baby desperately wanting to suck and swallow to try to relieve the acid heartburn.

○ Will take only small feeds: the baby very quickly learns that the more feed he takes in one go, the more pressure is put on the LOS and he starts to reflux.

○ Complete refusal of feeds: often due to the rapid association a baby makes between feeding and experiencing discomfort and pain.

○ Infrequent bowel movements, or showing great distress when straining to pass a stool: due to the internal pressure causing the stomach contents to reflux when passing a bowel motion. In fact, many babies will often poo only while feeding, as swallowing helps to wash down the acid that refluxes into the oesophagus as they strain to pass a motion.

○ Constipation or very hard, 'solid' stools: often associated with a cow's-milk protein intolerance.

- Explosive, very loose, watery, mucous and often green stools: can be associated with a lactose intolerance.
- No interest in feeds, doesn't naturally 'root' and look for feeds, fails to wake for feeds and refuses to latch on properly to the breast or gags if given a bottle within the first few days after birth: can be a very early indication that the baby is already suffering some degree of discomfort from acid reflux.
- Bouts of gagging and choking: due to vomit, along with some acid, refluxing up the oesophagus and hitting the back of the throat.
- Excessive dribbling: caused by the body producing extra saliva, which is a natural antacid and helps to combat the overproduction of the stomach acid.
- Appears to fall asleep after a few minutes' feeding and is impossible to wake to continue with the feed: I call this 'shut-down' and believe it to be a baby's self-defence mechanism kicking in when he does not want to take any more feed because he knows it is going to cause him pain.
- Cries when laid horizontal: when a baby is put on his back the LOS is somewhat stretched and opens more easily, therefore allowing the acid to reflux into the oesophagus and so causing severe heartburn. This is the same reason that, when laid on his back to sleep, a baby may cry with pain from the heartburn and be unable to sleep.
- Does not sleep well: due to general discomfort from the reflux. When he stirs throughout his sleep cycles he is often too uncomfortable to settle himself back to sleep.
- Very noisy, grunting and groaning, and will often even cry out when asleep: due to the pain of reflux and heartburn.
- Poor weight gain or failure to thrive: due to the development of a food aversion as he knows it causes pain.
- Normal growth and weight gain, but shows other symptoms: many babies do have an acceptable weight gain and appear to thrive, but this is often down to the instinctive perseverance and diligence of a mother to nurture and feed her baby whatever it takes.
- Excessive weight gain and wanting to feed and suckle all the time: some babies don't make the distinction between pain and hunger and instinctively look for food as a comfort.

○   Wants to be constantly held and will rarely settle if not being cuddled or carried in a baby-sling: the upright position assists natural gravity, which helps to keep the stomach contents in place.

○   Will sleep only when being held in a parent's arms: the comfort he feels can help to deal with his discomfort and pain. Also, being upright, as mentioned in the previous point, often gives some relief.

○   Having excess mucus and seeming to have a continual cold: due to the sinuses producing extra mucus in response to the presence of the stomach acid in the oesophagus, throat and nasal passages.

○   Constant cough or raspy breath: again due to the presence of acid in the oesophagus and throat, and to the extra mucus that is produced to try to negate this acid, which in turn causes a constant cough, often exacerbated when the baby is put on his back.

○   Grimacing or often frowning: I often think that a baby can look like a worried little old man when he is dealing with the effects of acid reflux.

○   Constantly clenches his fists and you may even find it difficult to prise them open – this is in reaction to his pain as he continually tries to deal with the pain from acid reflux.

○   Rarely smiles, seems withdrawn and is very quiet: all the baby's focus and concentration is on dealing with his discomfort.

○   Foul-smelling breath: due to the reflux of acid and part-digested milk.

○   Sore lips and mouth: caused when the acid burns not only the oesophagus internally but externally the lips and skin around the mouth.

○   Oesophagitis: damage caused to the oesophagus by continual contact with the refluxed acid; sometimes leads to severe burns and the development of ulcers.

○   Gagging himself with fingers or fist: often due to oesophagitis caused by the acid (see previous point).

Less common symptoms and causes include:

○   Tendency to bouts of infant apnoea (stops breathing) either during feeding or when asleep: this is possibly an extreme of the 'shut-down' scenario mentioned earlier (see page 210) due to severe pain.

○ Frequent ear infections or sinus congestion often developing as the baby gets older: due to the constant overproduction of mucus and from acid damage and scar tissue forming in the Eustacian tubes that lead into the ear.

○ Prone to aspirate when being sick: occurs when a baby breathes and inhales the vomit and/or milk into his lungs. Best described as a shocked, sharp and sudden intake of breath caused as the acid and vomit travel up an already sore and ulcerated oesophagus.

○ Respiratory problems, recurrent pneumonias, bronchitis, wheezing and asthma: due to continual aspiration and acid damage.

○ Erosion of dental enamel: due to the acid attacking the teeth.

○ Anaemia: due to constant vomiting and the malabsorption of feeds.

As you can see, the list is endless and I have yet to come across a baby who displays all these symptoms – in fact, it's a near impossibility. The facts that the range is so vast and the symptoms vary so dramatically from one baby to another are the main reasons why the understanding and diagnosis of reflux are extremely difficult.

Of course, some babies may display one or two of the above symptoms but on the whole are healthy, feeding and sleeping well, and may be nothing more than just a little unsettled at times. However, for those babies who are experiencing more than a few symptoms and are rarely able to feed or sleep comfortably then you should seek further help through a GP, health visitor, paediatrician or an expert in the field (known as a paediatric gastroenterologist). Some of you, though – because of your local health professionals perhaps not having much knowledge or a full understanding of the condition – need to be prepared for a bit of a battle and to stand your ground until you find someone who does understand and will take you seriously.

Alison says . . .

Reflux is a medical condition which needs a proper diagnosis, with ongoing supervision, and the appropriate management and treatment to relieve the baby of his symptoms.

One of the main symptoms people associate with reflux is vomiting. The amount and frequency of any vomiting will vary greatly from baby to baby, day to day and feed to feed. Some babies will continually just spit up small mouthfuls of vomit throughout the day and night; some may be quite sick for some time after feeding; others may projectile-vomit, usually during or directly after a feed. Sometimes a baby will be sick with such force that the vomit is projected through not only the mouth but the nose as well. As you may imagine, this can be so alarming the first time it happens that it can induce huge panic and distress in both parents and baby. It is not unusual for vomit to come out of the nose because as it is pushed up the oesophagus with such force the soft palate at the back of the mouth is unable to close properly, which then allows the vomit to pass into both the mouth and the nasal passages at the same time. This can often be very painful for the baby, as the acid can burn the back of his throat and nasal passages. So, although this fairly common physiological occurrence is nothing to worry about in itself, continual episodes of vomiting by your baby or suspected reflux should be discussed with your GP or other medical professional.

In some cases vomiting may be the only symptom that your baby displays and he may not appear distressed by having reflux in any other way. If the vomiting is minimal and is managed with relative ease, then there is little cause for concern. However, if your baby is vomiting with any degree of force and this occurs more than a couple of times a day, it would be advisable to seek some medical help. In my experience, although the vomiting may seem insignificant during the early months, if it is not brought under control it can lead to your baby continuing to vomit when he gets older, as his gag reflex becomes oversensitive. The introduction of solid food can then become a real challenge. I have come across a number of older babies and toddlers who still refuse to eat solid foods, often gag on any lumps or lumpy food, appear not to be able to swallow and have even learned how to make themselves vomit as a behavioural protest!

If your baby is vomiting on a regular basis, then it is a good idea to keep a note of when it happens in relation to a feed, the content and consistency of the vomit, how often in 24 hours and how much vomit is produced. Do remember, though, that sick, like blood, always looks to be more than it really is. As a guide you can do a 'vomit-volume' test by measuring out 30ml (1 fluid ounce) of water and tipping it on to the floor or on to a muslin to see how much it appears to be. Many parents are convinced that their baby is throwing up nearly all his feed, but after doing my 'vomit-volume' test they realize that the amount being brought up is far less than they actually thought.

Keeping a diary not only of vomiting episodes but of all your baby's behaviour, symptoms, bouts of crying and sleep habits (or the lack of them) will prove to be an invaluable aid when trying to explain his condition to your doctor or paediatrician.

Silent reflux

The most common misconception related to reflux is that if a baby is not throwing up then he doesn't have reflux. This most misleading fact often leads to many cases of 'silent reflux' being ignored or misdiagnosed. 'Silent reflux' is the term most commonly used, but some people in the medical world use the term 'occult', which means 'hidden' reflux and I think this is a much better description of the condition, especially as babies who suffer from it are rarely silent!

This type of reflux is caused by the same physiological events as previously described, but instead of the reflux material being projected as vomit it fluctuates between the stomach and the throat, staying in the oesophagus before eventually subsiding back into the stomach. Babies who suffer from this type of reflux often experience severe pain because the acidic material stays in contact with the oesophagus and throat causing extreme heartburn. In many cases the acid damage can become chronic, causing the oesophagus to become extremely sore, inflamed and even ulcerated. As the stomach contents reflux up into the oesophagus it can often be audible: loud 'gurgling' and 'churning' noises may be heard along with any amount of grunting, groaning, coughing and spluttering – far from 'silent'.

Mum's the Word . . .

When my second baby arrived *nothing* had prepared me for what we were about to face. Having already had our baby girl and survived that experience relatively well, I was feeling much calmer about the arrival of our son, thinking it would be a breeze this time around. Ha! – how wrong can you be?

My baby was born screaming and basically never stopped for the next three months. I was even asked to keep him quiet in hospital that first night, as he was disturbing the others on the ward! I would have loved to have stopped him crying, but nothing I did worked. He cried before a feed, he cried during a feed and he cried after a feed – and of course he hardly ever slept.

I had been to the GP and health visitors countless times and was told it was colic, that he was just a 'screamer', but worst of all that it was my stress and anxiety that was causing his distress!

I had to hold my baby continually and was never able to put him down, which had such a negative impact on my little girl. She changed from her usual happy, independent self and became so upset and clingy that life was a complete nightmare. The day I caught sight of myself in the bathroom mirror while sat on the loo holding my crying son with my daughter climbing all over me, I knew I had to find some help and someone to listen.

Miraculously, through a friend of a friend I found Alison, who simply changed our lives. She diagnosed silent reflux, sent us to see her gastro-paed, helped us to understand our son's condition, how to manage it and then how to teach him to sleep through the night.

We have never looked back since and are so grateful that someone finally listened and understood – and knew that I was not just going mad!

E. P.

Sadly, I have witnessed too many babies suffering with untreated and undiagnosed silent reflux. Most of them just scream inconsolably when they suffer a bout. It is the most distressing thing in the world for parents to deal with, as there is very little that can be done to comfort these babies and they will often carry on screaming until the pain from the heartburn attack subsides.

Mum's the Word . . .

❧ Silent reflux is something I probably never would have found out about myself and life was becoming really hard with a baby who was seemingly going backwards in terms of sleeping patterns and general happiness. Although it was really tough for around three months while we assessed the problem and got on the right drugs, and most importantly helped Jack to learn and trust that he was OK, I now have a baby who sleeps beautifully and still has a very positive association to food and is becoming a very 'normal' baby once more. ❧

A. L.

As with babies who vomit, it is a really good idea to keep a diary to note the bouts of the screaming and crying. It will also help a doctor to understand what is actually happening if you play him a video recording of your baby as he experiences an attack. All too often when parents take their babies to yet another doctor's appointment, because of the distraction the baby will be all smiles and seem completely happy while in the surgery. Coupled with the facts that the baby outwardly seems healthy, has had a relatively good weight gain and the doctor does not actually witness a feed, which is the usual cause of a reflux attack, it becomes very difficult for the doctor to make a firm diagnosis. In fact, I have found that many mums who have a baby suffering from silent reflux are often themselves prescribed antidepressants as their health professionals misdiagnose the baby's symptoms as perhaps 'just a bit of colic' and believe the anxiety in the mother to be caused by post-natal depression rather than by the instinctive knowledge that there is something wrong with her baby.

Feeding a reflux baby

Whether a baby is vomiting with his reflux or not, feeding often becomes a very stressful and time-consuming focus of the day for many parents. It never ceases to amaze me how individual reflux babies can react so differently towards their feeds. Some babies struggle to differentiate between pain in the oesophagus and hunger pangs in the stomach, so they instinctively look for food all the time. Others quickly learn that sucking and swallowing will bring some temporary relief from the burning pain of having acid reflux and therefore try to eat as much as possible. For some, the comfort they get from following their natural, inborn instinct to suckle will override the physical feeling of pain they get from reflux as they eat, and therefore they will continually search for more and more food.

On the other hand, many babies will quickly make the association between taking a feed and then experiencing the discomfort of reflux and this causes them to build up an aversion to eating. Their natural instinct to 'root' for food and to feed at regular intervals can often be suppressed, causing them to refuse feeds completely or more commonly to take what seems like hours over each feed. For parents this can be a complete nightmare. A mother has a natural instinct to feed and nurture her baby, so it can be extremely frustrating and upsetting when a baby doesn't want to feed and fights against it all the way. Many of these babies have a very poor weight gain, which understandably fuels their parents' anxiety and worry. Sadly, I have seen too many cases where a baby will eventually refuse all feeds completely. It is vitally important that a baby never feels 'forced' into taking feeds, as this will only deepen his aversion, but that an early diagnosis is gained and the appropriate course of medication, milk, feed-management and routine is found and put in place.

Mum's the Word . . .

For the first four months my baby would demand a feed every hour or so round the clock and as long as I fed her this way she rarely cried, continued to sustain her growth percentile and appeared to be 'content' most of the time. However, after four months of no proper sleep both she and I were completely exhausted and the underlying problems really became evident when I tried to switch to bottlefeeding.

I called Alison for help and when she arrived she realized almost instantly that this was a severe case of silent reflux. Alison explained that my baby had learned to 'manage' her pain and discomfort by taking very small quantities of milk every hour or so. When we introduced the bottle she would take only 1–2 ounces and then she would start to rub her feet together violently, thrash her head, her hands and feet would become wet with sweat and she would refuse to take any more of the feed.

After introducing Losec Mups, she gradually started to drink more milk at each feed. It was absolutely fascinating to learn from Alison what my baby's behaviour had meant. I had no idea that the head-thrashing, etc., were signs of stress and discomfort. As the medication kicked in, my baby started to take more volume at each feed and it was amazing to see her go through the '2-ounce barrier', at which point her hands and feet would still get really sweaty and you could see the look of panic on her face. But she quickly realized it didn't cause her pain any longer and she was able to carry on taking the feed comfortably.

I now understand that most of the behaviour that my baby displays is her way of trying to tell me something – it's just difficult sometimes to read it right!

N. B.

Through feeding in a certain way, some babies even learn to 'manage' their symptoms for themselves to try to reduce their pain and discomfort. This can take many forms, but the most usual is for the baby to demand very small but frequent feeds as he quickly learns that taking more than a certain volume of milk at one time fills the stomach, puts pressure on the already weak oesophageal sphincter and leads to a bout of reflux. I have seen many babies feed in this way and outwardly seem to thrive, appearing happy and rarely crying, but as time passes the situation becomes completely unmanageable for the parents, who may be still feeding their six-month-old baby round the clock. Also, even though the baby appears to be content, he *will* be overtired, may be inwardly stressed, and will possibly start to lose weight and refuse solid food. It is quite often suggested that feeding 'little and often' is a good way to cope with a reflux baby, but the trouble is that this just masks the condition without actually solving it. If a baby is being breastfed in this way then his stomach is never properly emptied, the contents are not fully digested and he constantly tops up his tummy on the lactose-rich foremilk. All this only exacerbates the reflux, the baby never learns to take a full feed and he never learns to sleep for any length of time as he is always looking for food. The answer, of course, is to get an early diagnosis and treat the reflux accordingly so that you and your baby can settle into the feeding and sleeping pattern advised in the earlier chapters of this book.

Another factor often mentioned in relation to feeding a baby with reflux is positioning. Whether the baby is breast- or bottlefed, the usual advice is to keep him upright during and after a feed, or at least to feed him at an elevated angle, the theory being that gravity should help to keep the contents in the stomach rather than allowing them to reflux up into the oesophagus by laying him down. Of course I understand the logic behind this advice, but although it may be a help for some babies it can actually cause more problems for others. Many babies with reflux who have built up an aversion to being fed seem to associate the feeling of being held closely with the pain suffered while feeding, so they display a negative reaction immediately when they are held in the 'feeding position'.

I have discovered that bottlefed reflux babies will often feed better if they are made comfortable on a pillow or cushion, which is placed next to you on a sofa or in front of you if you are sitting on a bed or the floor.

Over time, I have come to realize that an important factor when feeding a reflux baby is that his body needs to be kept straight rather than being bent in the middle – for example, when being held in the crook of an arm – so that little or no pressure is applied to his abdomen. As long as the baby's body is kept fairly straight, you can experiment with the reclining level of the supporting pillow or cushion to discover which suits him the best. I have even come across some babies who will feed only while lying completely flat. Anyway, trying to keep a baby upright when giving a feed is actually quite tricky – and as the feeding-harness that suspends him from the ceiling has not yet hit the market, it remains almost an impossibility! (I hope this doesn't give anyone the urge to invent one!)

I also feel that some babies prefer to have the freedom to move their heads, arms and legs around as opposed to feeling restrained when held in your arms. I do understand that some parents have such difficulty in feeding a reflux baby that they resort to swaddling him to keep him still, but although this is acceptable during the very early weeks I would not advise it as a long-term solution. As babies develop they do need to feel that they have some sense of independence over their feeding habits and it is all too easy for parents to fall into the trap of almost restraining their baby to the point of force-feeding – albeit unintentionally – a baby who is failing to gain weight.

Trying to feed a reflux baby who refuses feeds or takes forever over a couple of ounces can easily become a highly stressful, emotionally charged and anxiety-filled experience. This may then result in the baby building up an even greater aversion to feed times. I really do appreciate that it can be extremely difficult, but do try to keep as calm and relaxed as possible, put on the radio or even the TV to lighten the atmosphere and don't fall into the 'entertaining trap' of using toys or other excessive distraction techniques to get through each feed. Sometimes babies with reflux will be so easily distracted during a feed that if something disturbs them or catches their attention they will break from feeding and then refuse to take any more. I have encountered many parents who become totally isolated as they choose to stay at home in order to give each feed in a really quiet, often darkened room with no distractions, and woe betide the person who enters the room, coughs or sneezes loudly or makes any sudden noise or movement that might distract the baby.

My best advice is to experiment with different feeding techniques and positions until you find the one that best suits both you and your baby. Just remember: there is no 'right' or 'wrong', and what works for one may not work for another.

Having a baby with reflux can become an isolating experience for many reasons, one of which is that because feeding times are so difficult, parents become reluctant to go out and feed their baby in public. Trying to contain or mop up volumes of vomit, or cope with a baby who is screaming in pain in front of others, is a daunting prospect. If you do find it too stressful to feed your baby in public, try to go out in between feed times as it is so important for you both to get some fresh air and a change of scene.

Breastfeeding and reflux

Breastfeeding can be quite tricky to get established at the best of times, as I have already explained in Chapter 2. If you have a baby suffering from any degree of reflux, it is likely to become even more of a challenge. I have helped many mums who have struggled for weeks to get their baby to breastfeed and it is only when reflux has eventually been diagnosed that they realize why they have had such great difficulty. As the intricacies of reflux are explained, these mothers begin to understand what their baby's behaviour has meant, the effect of this on their milk production and supply, and why it has been so hard to establish any sort of feeding routine.

We all know the saying 'breast is best', but actually I believe this is not always the case for some babies with reflux. I have read and understood all the theories supporting this statement, and on the whole it may be true, but through my work I have been unable to ignore the fact that sometimes breast is *not* best when dealing with this condition. I do understand that many mothers have a strongly emotional and deeply rooted desire to breastfeed and may feel devastated and inadequate if unable to do so or if faced with the prospect of having to give up. There are many different opinions on whether breastfeeding actually makes the symptoms of reflux easier for the baby to deal with, or whether breast milk can aggravate the symptoms. In truth, every case of reflux is different and all mothers and babies should be treated as individuals, with some babies responding well to breast milk whereas others do not. As long as you have obtained an early diagnosis and then gained an understanding of how to manage your baby's reflux, it may be possible still to breastfeed for as long as you wish.

Through my research, years of experience and a survey of over 100 reflux cases, I have compiled the following list of pros and cons with regard to breastfeeding a reflux baby.

Pros:
- Some reflux babies do find breast milk easier to digest than formula.
- In some cases reflux can lower the baby's immunity, so the antibodies in breast milk give this a natural boost.
- Nursing at the breast can be a comfort to a baby crying in pain from reflux.
- Some medics believe breast milk to be a natural antacid which may help to counteract the overproduction of stomach acid.
- Breastfeeding may be less time consuming, as milk is readily available day or night.
- Some babies are more likely to drink breast milk as they prefer the taste.
- Babies will rarely become constipated when breastfed, so the reflux symptoms may be reduced as there is less pressure in the bowel.

Cons:
- Breast milk is usually a fairly thin, almost watery liquid which is more easily refluxed. A thicker, heavier consistency of feed uses the natural aid of gravity and will be more likely to stay down.
- Trying to get a reflux baby to latch on to the breast and stay there for a whole feed is often extremely difficult. Nipples can then become very sore because the baby continually pulls on and off the breast.
- Once on the breast, after taking a small amount of milk babies can easily fall into the 'shutdown' mode that I have already mentioned on page 210. They can do this when bottlefeeding, but it is easier to rouse them when away from the warmth and comfort of the breast.

○ It is impossible to tell how much milk the baby has taken even though he appears to be feeding efficiently. This of course is true for all breastfeeding mums, but when a baby has reflux it is often only after a significant weight loss that anyone will realize there has been, and still is, a problem. As I have already explained, babies can easily mask their symptoms by seeming to be sucking and drinking well when in fact they are not swallowing much milk at all.

○ Leading on from the previous point, if a baby continues to take only small amounts from the breast at each feed, this will have the knock-on effect of the milk supply not being properly stimulated and the breasts getting used to producing only small amounts of milk at frequent intervals.

○ Some babies with reflux can be very sensitive to the changes in breast milk brought about by the mother's diet and can react to certain foods that she eats. She may then need to eliminate them from her diet, which can ultimately become fairly restrictive.

○ If a baby has a cow's-milk protein allergy or intolerance, the mother will need to adopt a dairy-free diet, which some mums will find hard to adhere to.

○ Many babies have a lactose intolerance which often makes the symptoms of reflux more severe. Breast milk has a high lactose content which cannot be reduced by dietary means, so if the baby's symptoms are severe, replacing breast milk with a lactose-free formula may be the only solution.

○ Some mothers may need to take medication during the lactation period and many drugs will undoubtedly pass into the breast milk and have an adverse effect on the baby, making the reflux much worse. Over the years I have discovered a link between lactating mothers taking prescribed antibiotics and the increase of the severity of the symptoms of reflux in their babies. In fact, in some cases the onset of a breastfed baby's reflux can be traced back to his mother taking antibiotics during pregnancy. The reflux symptoms often then continue even after the mother has finished the course of tablets, because the action of the antibiotics that passed through the breast milk can strip the lining of the stomach which changes the pH balance, strips the healthy 'gut-flora' and increases the acidity. This can then lead to the baby quickly building up an intolerance to milk and he will need to be fed with one of the hypo-allergenic formulas explained on pages 226–30.

Some mothers may find that actual breastfeeding is not working for them or their baby and then may decide to express their milk and feed through a bottle rather than introducing a formula. This can prove to be quite time consuming and some mothers do find it to be unsustainable as a long-term option. However, the benefits can be that you can monitor the baby's intake more accurately, the nutritional benefits of breast milk are still provided and any medicated feed thickeners can be added to the breast milk before feeding.

As with any baby, reflux or not, if at any point you want the option of using a bottle for one or more feeds here or there, then it is best to introduce this within the first few weeks, thus avoiding a complete rejection by the baby of the bottle in favour of the breast at any stage. Reflux babies can be very difficult to feed at the best of times, are extremely sensitive to any change in their feeding habits and can be even more resistant to the introduction of a bottle.

Bottlefeeding and reflux

Many babies who become difficult to feed are often suffering from undiagnosed acid reflux, but initially the parents can wrongly assume that the type of bottle or teat that they are using is causing the problem. I have seen so many cupboards filled with an assortment of different bottles, teats, sippy cups, etc. – even bottles made as imitation breasts! – which the parents have tried in desperation, but all to no avail as the design of bottle and/or teat is rarely what is causing the problem. Swapping brands or types of bottle rarely makes any difference – it is the reflux that needs to be diagnosed, treated and managed before the baby will be able to feed more comfortably.

However, the size of the teat can make a slight difference and you will need to experiment with slow-, medium- or fast-flow teats to find which is most suitable for your baby. Some babies prefer to feed at a slow pace and will feel overwhelmed by a faster flow, whereas others seem to have a desire to drink the milk as quickly as possible and easily become frustrated if the flow is too slow. Many babies with reflux quickly learn how to 'pretend' that they are drinking and only when you break the feed do you see that hardly any milk has been taken. If your baby has developed this tactic, then you will need to concentrate on his feeds and watch closely to see if he is swallowing or not. There are many ways you can try to encourage him to continue feeding while he is still latched on to the bottle, such as tickling his chin or stroking his cheek, twisting or gently tugging on the bottle, gently blowing on his face, tickling his feet, moving his arms up and down, and even sprinkling drops of water on his face.

If your doctor has prescribed Infant Gaviscon or suggested using a feed-thickener such as Instant Carobel, then a 'Y'-cut or variable-flow teat may be necessary. Likewise, some of the ready-thickened formulas like Stay Down or Enfamil AR will often clog a standard-holed teat but flow much more freely from those teats designed for thicker liquids.

Most babies suffering from acid reflux can become highly sensitive, especially to anything and everything related to their feeds. I have known some refuse warm milk, taking it only once it has cooled down, while others appear to feed better if the milk is kept at a warmer temperature. When feed time can take over an hour this may prove difficult, so some mums resort to having a bottle warmer always to hand – but over time this becomes quite restrictive. If it does become a problem, my advice is to try to gradually lower the temperature of the milk over the space of a week or so until the baby will accept it at room temperature. If you choose to bottlefeed right from the start and offer only feeds at room temperature, then your baby will not know anything different.

How you position your baby can also make a big difference when bottlefeeding, as explained above (see pages 217–21). Further to this, always try to ensure that the baby's head is tilted back rather than with the chin towards the chest as this keeps the throat more open, allowing the milk to flow freely and reducing the chance of a gag-reflex. You may find it useful to re-read the 'positioning' section in Chapter 2 (see pages 40–43).

Formulas

There are many different formulas available and some are designed specially for babies suffering with acid reflux, cow's-milk protein and/or lactose intolerances or allergies. The type of formula that is best for your baby will depend on his individual symptoms and should always be discussed with your doctor. Always follow the manufacturers' guidelines when using any formula for your baby.

As with introducing or changing any medications, it is important not to try too many new things at once as it is then difficult to tell what works and what doesn't. When switching to a new or different formula, do make sure that enough time is allowed for the previous milk to leave the system completely and for the new one to be accepted before assessing whether the change has produced a positive response or not. Sometimes, if moving from a dairy formula on to a hydrolysed one, the baby may reject the new formula because of its taste. If this happens, then it may take time to wean the baby gradually on to the new milk by mixing this with the existing milk, increasing the strength ratio each day. For example, the following tables show how to wean from either expressed breast milk or Aptamil on to Nutramigen:

Day	Water	Aptamil	Nutramigen
Day 1	180ml (6 fl. oz)	5 scoops	1 scoop
Day 2	180ml (6 fl. oz)	4 scoops	2 scoops
Day 3	180ml (6 fl. oz)	3 scoops	3 scoops
Day 4	180ml (6 fl. oz)	2 scoops	4 scoops

Day	Water	Aptamil	Nutramigen
Day 5	180ml (6 fl. oz)	1 scoop	5 scoops
Day 6	180ml (6 fl. oz)	–	6 scoops

Day	Expressed breast milk	Water	Nutramigen
Day 1	150ml (5 fl. oz)	30ml (1fl. oz)	1 scoop
Day 2	120ml (4 fl. oz)	60ml (2 fl. oz)	2 scoops
Day 3	90ml (3 fl. oz)	90ml (3 fl. oz)	3 scoops
Day 4	60ml (2 fl. oz)	120ml (4 fl. oz)	4 scoops
Day 5	30ml (1 fl. oz)	150ml (5 fl. oz)	5 scoops
Day 6	–	180ml (6 fl. oz)	6 scoops

> ### *Alison says . . .*
>
> The quicker you can instigate the change on to the dairy/
> lactose-free formula, the better. First try offering a full-strength
> bottle of the new, hydrolized formula. If your baby refuses,
> you could then try making the switch in just 3 days by using a
> stronger ratio each day.

The following list explains the formulas most commonly advised or prescribed. Medical advice should always be sought when introducing formula to your baby's diet.

- Ordinary cow's milk-based formulas such as Aptamil, SMA, etc., may be suitable if the baby has little or no cow's-milk protein/lactose intolerance or allergy. Infant Gaviscon or other feed thickeners can be added to these milks.
- Formulas like Easy Digest and Comfort are nearly always cow's-milk-based but have a reduced lactose content and are usually of a thicker consistency when made up. They are designed to relieve mild reflux symptoms and may need to be fed through a faster-flow teat.
- There are a couple of Stay Down formulas on the market which also are dairy-based but have added rice- or cornstarch to make them thicker and more satisfying. The idea behind this is that if the baby feels full more quickly he will need to take less volume, which may reduce the chance of a reflux attack. There is some concern, though, that the baby's essential nutrition may be at risk if the formula is bulked out with starch supplements and does not provide sufficient nutrients.
- Some brands of general formula offer lactose-free alternatives (e.g. SMA LF) designed for those babies who can tolerate cow's-milk protein but have a lactose intolerance.
- Enfamil AR is a cow's-milk-based formula that is pre-thickened with a rice starch. This formula is fluid when made up but thickens in the baby's stomach as it reacts with the gastric juices. It can be quite

effective for some babies who are prone to vomiting.

○ Enfamil O-Lac is basically the same as Enfamil AR but has had the lactose removed, making it suitable for babies with reflux who also have a lactose intolerance.

○ Nutramigen is a hypo-allergenic formula used for babies with either a cow's-milk protein and/or lactose intolerance. The protein in it has been extensively broken down (hydrolysed) into tiny pieces that are not recognized by the immune system and will not trigger an allergic reaction in most babies. Nutramigen 1 is for babies up to six months and Nutramigen 2 for those six months and older.

○ Nutramigen AA is an amino-acid-based formula for babies with a severe cow's-milk protein allergy and those who may not tolerate an extensively hydrolysed formula. The protein has been completely broken down into amino acids which make for easy digestion.

○ Neocate is a similar formula to Nutramigen AA and is designed for babies with a severe cow's-milk protein allergy and/or multiple food-protein intolerances. Elemental ingredients are broken down into the purest form for easy digestion. It also contains 'free' amino acids which are man-made rather than coming from animal or soya protein and so are less likely to cause a reaction.

○ Pregestimil is a formula for babies who have a problem with digestion or absorption of routine formulas, or who are diagnosed with cow's-milk protein allergy and fat malabsorption. It is lactose- and sucrose-free and the carbohydrate is readily digested and well tolerated as it contains a special fat called MCT (medium chain triglycerides) oil which is easily absorbed and shown to promote weight gain in babies with fat malabsorption and who may be failing to thrive.

○ Soya-based milks are marketed as an alternative to dairy formulas, but their long-term use is not usually recommended. The protein contained in soya milk can build up over time in the baby's system, causing him to develop an allergic reaction to it. It can be a useful short-term alternative when a break from the usual cow's-milk-based formula is advised due to a bout of illness such as gastro-enteritis or bronchiolitis (RSV).

○ Infatrini is dairy-based, high-calorie, concentrated formula designed for babies who are struggling to gain weight.

○ Dou-Cal is a high-calorie nutritional supplement that can be added to other formulas to help babies who are struggling to gain weight.

Lactose intolerance

Lactose intolerance is the inability to digest significant amounts of lactose, which is the major sugar found in milk. People sometimes confuse lactose intolerance with cow's-milk protein intolerance because the symptoms can be very similar. However, they are not related and are two separate conditions. A cow's-milk allergy or intolerance is a reaction triggered by the immune system, whereas lactose intolerance is a problem caused by the digestive system.

Mum's the Word . . .

Logan did nothing but sleep as a baby. He drank very well but could then projectile the whole bottle at least twice a day. Our worry was that he was so quiet and had little interest in the outside world. Alison observed that he appeared to be struggling to digest his food and had rancid, lumpy-green nappies. We switched his feed to a lactose-free formula and he completely changed. He smiled at us on the first day of his new formula, and although he was still quite a sicky baby he became a happy, alert little boy – nothing like the unhappy, withdrawn little soul we took home from hospital. He also adapted to Alison's plan really well and slept through the night at six weeks.

K. B.

Lactose intolerance is fairly common in babies and is due to a shortage of the enzyme lactase in an immature digestive system. Lactase is needed to break down the lactose in milk and if it is deficient the baby may suffer from excess and/or trapped wind, bloating of the abdomen, explosive stools which are often green and watery, and stomach cramps. Many premature babies will suffer with a lactose intolerance because lactase levels do not increase until into the third trimester of a woman's pregnancy. Generally, babies will outgrow the lactose intolerance as their digestive system develops, but in rare cases there can be a more serious underlying cause, such as Crohn's disease, Coeliac disease or inflammatory bowel disease.

To test for a lactose intolerance your doctor may carry out the 'stool acidity test' which will detect the presence of any lactic acid, which is created by bacteria in undigested lactose. However, if the baby is already being formula-fed, a simpler option is to switch to a lactose-free alternative to see if the symptoms lessen. For breastfed babies it is not quite so simple, as it is impossible to remove the lactose from the mother's breast milk. A product called Colief – a synthetic form of the enzyme lactase – is available and, when given before each feed, can help to break down the lactose in the milk and may reduce the symptoms a little. For some babies with a severe lactose intolerance it may be necessary to replace breast milk completely with a lactose-free alternative formula.

Cow's-milk protein (dairy) intolerance and allergy

Some babies have an intolerance to the protein in cow's milk. This can cause them to be generally unsettled and they may be constipated or have loose, runny stools. It can induce vomiting or continual spit-up of feeds, eczema-type dry and sore patches on the skin, and is often a major factor in cases of reflux. Some babies I have seen appear puffy and bloated with their skin feeling quite clammy and this, I have discovered, can also be related to a dairy intolerance.

For babies who are breastfed it will be necessary to remove all dairy products from the mother's diet, ensuring that they are replaced by suitable supplements. It may be advisable to seek professional advice from a dietician on how best to achieve this. If the baby is already formula-fed, then a change to a specialized dairy-free formula would be advisable.

In some cases babies actually have an allergy to the cow's-milk protein and will display some or all of the symptoms already mentioned, but these can be much more severe and sometimes result in an anaphylactic shock reaction which can prove extremely serious.

Generally speaking, children usually outgrow their intolerances and most allergic reactions subside by around three years of age.

Medications and diagnostic tests

Antacids

Simple antacids are usually used as the first line of treatment when reflux is diagnosed. The most common antacid used in the UK is Infant Gaviscon and this medication can often give babies some immediate relief. However, it may seem to work well for a couple of days but then seem to wear off and the symptoms return. This is due to the amount of acid reflux being more severe than Gaviscon alone can deal with, so a stronger acid-blocker may also be required. This type of medication, although it can work quickly, does not have a long-lasting effect as it only neutralizes the stomach acid immediately after being taken, which is why it needs to be given with each feed.

Gaviscon can help to reduce the burning sensation in the oesophagus and also to thicken the contents of the stomach, so reducing the backward flow of reflux.

As stated by the manufacturer, constipation can be a side-effect of Gaviscon, as some babies react to its aluminium content. More often than not, however, it can help to keep the bowels regular as it contains magnesium, which acts as a laxative. When Gaviscon is introduced it may initially change the regularity of the bowel movements, while the consistency of the stools does become more solid. However, after the first couple of motions have been passed and the baby's system adapts to the change, all should normalize fairly quickly.

Gaviscon is often a useful medication when treating reflux, but in my experience it can be very difficult to administer according to the manufacturer's directions. The advice is to make it up with 15ml (0.5 fl. oz) of water and give it after a feed, but it can be almost impossible to get such a volume of medication into a reflux baby who has already taken his quota of feed. Also, I have often found that giving any medication on top of a feed will just make the baby vomit. The instructions also state that the powder can be added to a formula feed, but all too often this will just clog up the teat and restrict the flow of milk.

Through my experience of using Infant Gaviscon I have found that the easiest ways to achieve the best results are:

○ For fully breastfed babies, use either one or two sachets, according to the stated dosage for your baby's age and weight. Put the Gaviscon powder into a small, clean pot and add 5ml of just-boiled water. Mix it into a syrup, dissolving all the lumps, draw it up into a 5ml syringe and give this to your baby directly before starting the feed. For best effect, Gaviscon needs milk with which to react and create the 'gel' that coats the oesophagus, neutralizes the acid and thickens the milk in the stomach, so feed your baby immediately after giving the dose.

○ If feeding expressed breast milk through a bottle, make up the dose of Gaviscon as explained above, then add the dose to the bottle of already warmed milk and feed immediately.

○ When using formula there are two ways of adding the Gaviscon to the feeds. The first is to make up the dose as previously explained and add the syrup to the made-up feed. Alternatively, you can mix the Gaviscon powder with the powdered milk as you add it to the water. I have found that if you just add the Gaviscon powder to any already made-up milk, no amount of shaking or stirring will get rid of the lumps and it will then clog up the teat. However, if you are using a 'Y'-cut or variable-flow teat this may not be a problem.

Alison says . . .

I always remind parents that reflux is rarely 'cured' by the use of medication, formulas and feed thickeners. The symptoms are only ever brought under control and the condition can only be 'managed' until the baby grows out of it.

Acid-blockers (H2 blockers)

These types of drugs work by blocking acid production and they usually take effect within three to six days. The body naturally produces the chemical histamine and one of its uses is to bind with the H2 receptors in the stomach lining which induces acid production to aid digestion. In cases of reflux the excess acid causes much pain and discomfort. An acid-blocker such as Ranitidine will stop the histamine from binding with the H2 receptors and will therefore reduce the acid production.

This medication is given in a weight-related dosage and its use should be monitored to allow for the baby's growth.

Motility agents

These drugs are known as Prokinetics and they work by speeding up the movement of food through the digestive system. In many reflux babies there is thought to be some degree of gastroparesis, or a delayed gastric emptying, so the chance of a reflux attack may be lessened by the use of these medications. The two most commonly used in the UK are:

○   Domperidone. This is a motility agent which, by helping to move food faster through the oesophagus, stomach and intestines, ensures that it doesn't stay too long in the same place or flow backwards. I have found that some babies do not sleep as restfully when taking this medication. It is possible that because the food moves through the gut more quickly they may feel more hungry, or that their system is forced to work overtime by the drug and therefore they become slightly more agitated and unable to rest or relax properly.

○ Erythromycin. This is an antibiotic which has the side-effect of increasing gastric motility. When given in low doses over an extended period it helps to increase the rate of digestion.

Proton pump inhibitors (PPIs)

In my opinion these are the most effective medications for treating acid reflux. All babies will respond differently to medications and some will have an immediate reaction to the introduction of a PPI, with some parents extolling it as a 'wonder drug', while for others it can take seven to ten days for its effect to become apparent. Taking the latter point into consideration, in some cases it is important to have a crossover period when switching from using one drug, such as Ranitidine, on to using a PPI.

PPIs work by almost totally shutting down the acid pumps in the stomach, which then reduces the gastric acid secretion by over 90 per cent.

Losec Mups (Omeprazole) is one of the most widely used drugs in the UK and comes in the form of a dispersible tablet. However, its use is not currently licensed for babies under a year old, although it is often prescribed 'off licence' at the discretion of a paediatrician or GP.

As this medication is 'off licence' there are no instructions in the patient information leaflet on how to administer it to infants under twelve months. Through my work with many hundreds of reflux babies, and having taken advice from various quarters, I have worked out that the easiest and most effective way to administer Losec to achieve optimum results is as follows:

○ When a Losec tablet is put in water it does not completely dissolve, with the result that the end solution is full of sediment and tiny granules which will easily block up a syringe. The tablet has a pinky-orange coating which does dissolve.

> ### *Alison says . . .*
>
> A client rang me in panic one day as her baby's·vomit appeared to be full of tiny red and black bits that looked like raspberry seeds. I now remember to warn every parent whose baby is taking Losec that this is quite normal as the grains from the tablet do not actually dissolve, but turn a dark shade of red after reacting with gastric acid and stay in the stomach for up to 20 hours.

- There is a very wide dosage scale in relation to weight, starting at 0.3mg and ranging upwards to 2.2mg per kilo of body weight.
- When Losec is prescribed for babies it usually comes in 10mg tablets. The easiest and most accurate doses can be given in multiples of 5mg, as each 10mg tablet can be snapped in half before dissolving. The tablets are quite soft and easy to snap in half, but make sure your hands are completely dry.
- To dissolve, use cooled, previously boiled water.
- Use two small pots (I use the caps from Avent bottles), putting the Losec tablet in one and some water in the other.
- Draw up 3ml of water into a syringe and gently squirt it on to the Losec, then wait a few minutes for it to disperse. The best syringes to use can be from packs of Infant Nurofen, Dentinox Colic Drops or a 1ml syringe from the chemist, as these have wider holes and block less easily.
- Once the tablet has dispersed, while continually agitating the suspension, gradually draw it up into the syringe.
- Hold the syringe in the palm of your hand, using your fingers to keep the syringe in place and your thumb at the end ready to depress the plunger. Keep turning your wrist back and forth to agitate the suspension continually and stop the sediment from settling.
- Have your baby on a flat, secure surface (his changing table is often best) so that you have both hands free.

○ If your baby is reluctant to open his mouth, use the thumb and forefinger of your other hand and apply slight pressure to both cheeks to ease his mouth open.

○ Place the end of the syringe in your baby's mouth and aim towards the back of either cheek.

○ Depress the plunger to give a small amount and keep repeating this until the syringe is empty.

○ Remember to keep agitating and turning the syringe between squirts.

○ Tip a tiny bit more water into the tablet pot and rinse round, draw it up into the syringe and repeat the administration to ensure that the complete dose, or as much as is possible, is given.

○ Some babies will cough, gag and splutter when given this medication. Try not to panic, but do persevere with its administration as the results for most babies with reflux are worth the battle.

○ Losec should not be given at the same time as a feed, as milk hinders its effectiveness.

○ Initially, it actually needs acidic conditions to take effect. Therefore if your baby struggles with the taste of the Losec, you can use diluted fruit juice instead of plain water when making up the medication. After the introduction of solids, it can be helpful to give the made-up suspension in a few spoonfuls of fruit purée.

○ Losec can be given either once a day or twice a day as a split dose. For example, sometimes a prescribed dose of 10mg in each 24 hours can be given as a half tablet (5mg) in the morning and the other half in the evening.

○ The morning dose is best given 30 minutes before either the first or second feed of the day. The evening dose is best given before bathtime, thus leaving 30 minutes before giving the bedtime feed.

○ Losec is usually started as a four-week course but, after monitoring the results, its use may be continued for longer.

○ After using this type of medication for any length of time it should never be withdrawn without an extended weaning-off period.

○ Once the symptoms of reflux are brought under control, it can be difficult to tell whether the condition itself has improved and the medication is no longer necessary. The only way to test this is gradually to lower the daily dose and continue with its withdrawal if all remains well, but reinstate the dose if the symptoms recur.

Some paediatricians opt to use a prescription of Omeprazole solution, assuming that it is easier to give to a baby than the dispersible tablet form. This, however, is not stocked as a medication, takes at least 48 hours to be prepared by the pharmacist, has a very unpleasant taste and a maximum shelf-life of twenty-one days. Furthermore, its effectiveness often wears off after fourteen days and it is extremely expensive, costing over £200 per 100ml bottle. Following my experiences in dealing with both these forms of Omeprazole, my conclusion is that Losec Mups is by far the better option.

Diagnosing reflux

In most cases a diagnosis of reflux is made according to the parent's explanation and description of the baby's symptoms. It is not usually necessary to carry out any diagnostic tests, as the symptoms alone should be enough to determine the condition. However, there are some cases that need further investigation, perhaps because they do not respond to the usual path of treatment or because there appear to be other complications. There are also certain conditions – pyloric stenosis or Coeliac disease, for example – that present with similar symptoms to reflux but are far more serious and need to be ruled out.

There are four main tests that can be carried out to confirm a reflux diagnosis and rule out other complications:

1) pH study
2) barium swallow
3) reflux scan
4) upper endoscopy

Your paediatrician will provide more information if any of these tests is deemed necessary. There are also various surgical procedures that can be carried out to control the most severe cases of GORD, but because of complications that can accompany this surgery it is only ever undertaken as a last resort and it is much too complex a subject to be included in this book. Likewise, there are some babies who suffer from severe reflux which is related to other more serious genetic or medical conditions which, sadly, I do not have space to cover here.

Sleeping and reflux

As I have already mentioned, many babies with GORD will struggle to sleep comfortably and are often disturbed throughout their sleep by acid heartburn. It is almost impossible to expect a baby who is suffering from any degree of reflux to be able to sleep soundly for any length of time, let alone through the night, until his symptoms have been treated and brought under control. Once a diagnosis has been given and the baby is responding to his path of treatment it will be easier to follow the Sensational Baby Sleep Plan as set out at the beginning of this book, or for older babies to implement the reassurance sleep-training technique explained in Chapter 6.

In my experience – and as I have already said many times throughout this book – sleep position can make a huge difference to the quality of a baby's sleep, especially if he has reflux. I have found very few reflux babies who are able to sleep comfortably, if at all, on their backs, whereas they greatly benefit from sleeping on their sides or even their fronts. When a baby lies on his back the lower oesophageal sphincter is more likely to relax and allow the valve it surrounds to flop open, thus allowing the stomach contents to reflux into the oesophagus. If the baby is on his side, then this is less likely to happen as the valve is kept partially closed; and if a baby is on his tummy, the pressure from lying on his front keeps the valve almost completely closed, preventing any reflux episodes. I appreciate that this is contrary to current sleeping-position guidelines, but in my view any baby with suspected or diagnosed reflux should have either a portable breathing and movement monitor fitted to his nappy 24/7 and/or an under-mattress breathing monitor in his cot, both of which will sound if the baby stops breathing no matter what his sleep position (see also Chapter 3). Sadly, I know of too many reflux babies who have had severe apnoea attacks or have aspirated on their own vomit, and some who have actually died as a result. As babies with reflux are at greater risk of this happening, and therefore at greater risk of cot death, my advice is to use one of these monitors as soon as reflux is suspected or diagnosed and this will mean the importance of sleeping your baby only on his back is much reduced.

Mum's the Word

Our baby girl was born in December 2008 and was given a clean bill of health upon our discharge from hospital. We were overjoyed with our baby, but as we settled in at home I began to feel a sense of unease. I was trying to breastfeed with little success and our baby girl seemed so unhappy and screamed most of the time. Being an older mum, I was fully aware that the route into parenthood would not be easy, but nothing prepared me for the distress we all felt.

I battled on and continually sought help from my local health visitors and GP, but all to no avail. I was told she was healthy and that maybe she just had colic. Then, when she had just turned four weeks old, I fed her as usual one afternoon and afterwards put her down into the carrycot next to me on the sofa. I turned away for a minute and when I looked back at Elin, she was turning blue and had obviously stopped breathing. I can't begin to describe my panic and fear, but as I scooped her up into my arms, thankfully she started breathing again.

We then spent the next week in hospital, where they carried out numerous different tests and sent us home with no diagnosis, but again just a clean bill of health.

I persevered with trying to find some answers, as the feeding was no better and the bouts of screaming were escalating. Finally, at eight weeks, it was suggested that she might have reflux and she was started on some low-dose antacid. At twelve weeks we saw Dr Eltumi, and after his confirmation of reflux and further medication Elin's symptoms were slowly brought under control.

We contacted Alison at four months and enlisted her help to redress Elin's feeding aversion and to help teach her to sleep.

Sadly, Elin's story is far too common and, as Alison pointed out, if I had not been next to Elin and noticed her turning blue the day she stopped breathing then she could have become another cot-death statistic. If Elin had been left in her carrycot for 10 minutes or more she might have just died there and then, but there would have been nothing to explain why. As Alison has explained, a baby with severe acid reflux can stop breathing at any time due to the sudden pain caused as acid comes up into the oesophagus. The baby's instinctive reaction causes a very sharp inhalation of breath which closes off the airways – classically known as an apnoea attack. But of course if a baby then does not start to breathe again and tragically slips away, there is no evidence to be found of the cause of death.

We have stayed in touch with Alison and her advice and help have been invaluable and her knowledge of babies neverending.

We are so lucky to have Elin with us today and I hope this story, alongside Alison's advice, helps to save other babies who may be at risk.

L. M.

I have been directly involved with a few families whose babies have actually stopped breathing and needed immediate medical attention. Some of these apnoea attacks occurred during the day, either during or shortly after a feed, and others occurred during sleep. All these instances were linked to severe, undiagnosed and therefore untreated cases of reflux and I believe that many unexplained infant deaths can be attributed to this condition.

In some cases it can be helpful to raise the head end of the cot or Moses basket so that your baby is lying at a slightly inclined angle. This is relatively easy to achieve while your baby is small and stays in one place, but as soon as he starts to wriggle around you may find he ends up in a heap at the bottom of the cot, which is not particularly safe, so you may then need to lower it again. Do make sure that you raise the head end of the whole cot or Moses basket using blocks or sturdy books; don't just prop up the head part of the mattress as this could mean that the baby is actually lying in a bent position rather than on a flat surface. Recently on sale in the UK is a 45-degree wedge-pillow with a body-harness attached into which the baby is strapped to keep him in an elevated sleep position, but so far I have not seen them used with much success and have found that babies can feel quite insecure when using them. However, I have found the 'side-sleep' positioning wedges to be quite useful in keeping a baby on his side without him being able to roll on to his back or his front.

All babies, but especially those with reflux, can be quite noisy while asleep. Reflux babies are known to groan and moan, cough and snuffle, writhe and wriggle, and can be generally restless throughout the night. Many parents find it almost impossible to sleep themselves when listening to their little refluxer all night and it may be easier to put the baby in his own room, using an under-mattress breathing sensor for peace of mind.

Inevitably, babies with reflux will cry more and be harder to settle down to sleep, but once the baby is more comfortable through treatment, the crying should subside. I have seen and heard many babies who cry out during sleep and can cry for a few minutes but will then re-settle. Parental instinct is to rush immediately to comfort the crying baby, especially when he has been suffering with the pain of reflux, but sometimes it is best to leave him for a few minutes longer to see if he is able to settle himself back to sleep. Many parents ask for my help as they reach a stage when they feel that they just can't 'read' their baby any longer and struggle to know whether the crying is from pain, lack of sleep, hunger, etc., or whether maybe it has become a behavioural habit. This confusion, usually induced in parents by their own continual sleep deprivation when looking after a reflux baby, can often lead to a nightly ritual of:

❍   Baby cries. Cuddle him – he's in pain.

❍   I'm cuddling him. Baby's now screaming.

❍   Put him back to bed? He's still crying . . .

❍   Offer a feed. He takes just a little. What now?

❍   Put him back to bed. He settles – but only for 20 minutes.

❍   Try a dummy. He settles for an hour. Now screaming again. Is it pain?

❍   Try to comfort him. Nothing works – give another feed?

❍   Now Daddy tries to settle him. They sleep together for an hour. Crying again . . .

❍   Try leaving him? He cries for an hour.

❍   Into bed with us. He still cries on and off till morning . . .

I have used this example to try to highlight just how difficult interpreting a baby's cry can be, especially at night when it all sounds so much louder, feels so much more distressing and the lights on the sound monitor go from green to red at an alarming rate just to make you feel even worse! Coping with a baby crying from reflux day or night can be so difficult, and until the right path of treatment is found, sadly there may not be much relief for either parents or baby.

Reflux behaviour – reactive or habitual?

When a baby has reflux and suffers any degree of pain, he will learn to express his discomfort through various behavioural signals. By reading the 'Signs and symptoms' section of this chapter (pages 207–14) you will see that many of them are the behavioural signals that an individual baby learns in order to express his reaction to pain. Typically, he may arch his back, thrash his head from side to side, become rigid and really scream as he suffers an attack of acid reflux. Once the correct medication and feeding method have been found and he has become more comfortable, these behavioural signals should lessen. However, it is not usually as simple as just medicating the baby and expecting everything to become 'normal' overnight. Medication can take time to work, and weaning the baby on to a new milk will also be a gradual process, but more importantly it can take a while for the baby to realize that the pain and discomfort he once suffered are actually subsiding.

When suffering the pain of reflux, most babies will have become accustomed to using particular learned patterns of behaviour to express themselves, so even though the pain and discomfort have been reduced the baby will still revert to displaying the same behaviour at other times of stress – for example, teething, going down with a cough or cold, but mostly when he is overtired. I have had many parents ask me why their baby still appears to be suffering from the pain of reflux and continues to display the same behaviour, even though he is fully medicated and on the correct milk. This is often because many reflux babies will not have learned to sleep properly and sleep deprivation can make them so fractious that they will often show the same behavioural symptoms they learned to display through having reflux.

In my experience it is nearly always necessary to re-train the baby and teach him how to sleep through the night once his reflux symptoms have been brought under control, as this is not something that is usually rectified with medication alone. See Chapter 6, which explains how to implement my reassurance sleep-training technique.

Introducing solids for a reflux baby

This can be a complex issue for some, while other babies readily accept solid food and take to it with ease. There is no set path that suits each baby – it is very much trial and error to discover the best way forward. Although current guidelines state that solid food should not be introduced until six months, it is often advised to start reflux babies sooner than this as solid food can help to improve their symptoms. In fact, I have found that there is often a very small window of opportunity for introducing solid food to some reflux babies and it can easily be missed by waiting too long. In general, it is accepted that the introduction of solids can start at any time from sixteen weeks and, if necessary, should be discussed with the doctor or health professional who is managing your baby's reflux.

Obviously, though, if your baby is four months old, has been suffering for some time but has only recently been diagnosed with reflux, he is likely to have built up an aversion to anything new being introduced to his mouth and it will be necessary to wait until his symptoms have been brought under control. Sadly for many babies, it can take such a long time for a proper diagnosis of reflux to be made that, due to the ongoing suffering they have experienced, they may already have built up such a deep-rooted aversion to their milk that this negative attitude is carried forward when solid foods are introduced. This can then become a very slow and painstaking experience for both parents and baby and much patience will be needed.

Generally I have found babies with reflux to be more accepting of vegetables than of fruit. Fruit is quite acidic and almost instinctively some babies will not touch it as they seem to sense it will exacerbate their reflux. My advice is to offer baby rice as a first food, mixed up with some of the baby's usual milk, then gradually introduce other foods as a flavour to the baby rice, rather than giving spoonfuls of 'neat' vegetables or fruit, which can be quite harsh on a baby's tummy. Again, there is no hard and fast rule that applies to all reflux babies. Many have varying degrees of food intolerances and allergies which need to be taken into consideration when introducing solid food. The table below is only a very rough guide to which first foods to try and which to avoid.

Trafffic-light food table

Green: OK	Amber: Caution	Red: Danger
courgette	avocado	apple
melon	banana	blackberry
parsnip	blueberry	citrus fruit
pear	broccoli	onion
pumpkin	cabbage	pineapple
squash	carrot	raspberry
swede	cauliflower	strawberry
	leek	tomato
	mango	
	peach	
	pepper	
	spinach	
	sweet potato	

If using ready-prepared jars, packets or pouches, do make sure you read the ingredients list carefully as some brands of baby food have a high apple content, and if your baby is on a dairy-free diet you will also need to check that it contains no added milk products.

Some babies who have regularly vomited due to their reflux may find it difficult to tolerate any solid food without gagging, and it will be necessary to persevere with different textures and consistencies of food to find what works best. Many will tolerate only thin purées, while others may bypass that stage completely and move straight on to finger food.

Other babies who have suffered with long-term undiagnosed reflux can develop dysphagia, which means they actually have difficulty swallowing. This is caused by severe acid-damage to the throat and oesophagus which leaves scar tissue when it heals. Because the scar tissue is much thicker than the original linings, the passage becomes narrower, hindering the swallowing of solid and lumpy food. Hence babies will often gag and choke on any food that is thicker than a purée and, as they grow older, children can develop a fear of swallowing any lumps because they have learned that it makes them choke.

Due to the fact that a reflux baby may have quickly built up an association between pain and drinking milk, many parents feel that feeding during the first few months is a complete nightmare, a stressful experience dreaded by both them and their baby. Taking the next step of introducing solids may look like just another mountain to climb. However, in most cases introducing solids can be the start of an improvement in the baby's reflux, albeit often a very gradual one, and in time eating should become a more positive experience for the whole family.

Coming off medication and outgrowing reflux

There are no rules governing when your baby may be ready to come off his medication: it is impossible to predict when each individual baby will have outgrown his reflux enough for his symptoms to disappear. In my experience, though, the earlier reflux is diagnosed and treated, the sooner it seems to subside and the baby will be able to come off any medication, whereas the longer he has reflux that is left untreated, the longer he will have to stay on his medication because he seems to take longer to outgrow his reflux.

Whatever combination of medication your baby ends up taking, it is likely that he will be on it for a number of weeks, if not months. I usually advise that if all has been relatively stable for around six weeks, then it may be a good idea to start gradually reducing the dosage to see what happens. If there seems to be no adverse reaction, then you can continue with the gradual withdrawal of the medication; however, if any of the symptoms reappear then you should just reinstate the original dose strength and wait another four weeks before trying again. It is never advisable suddenly to stop giving any antacid medication that your baby has been on for some time, but always to wean him off it gradually. Your paediatrician should be able to give you more detailed advice on when your baby may be ready to come off his medication and will suggest a plan for its withdrawal.

☆ *Alison's Golden Rules* ☆

1   If you instinctively feel that there is something wrong, or not quite right, with your baby, trust your instincts and persevere with trying to find someone who will listen and be able to help.

2   Keep a diary recording some of your baby's feeds, sleeps, bouts of crying or vomiting and periods of being unsettled and take it with you to show your doctor.

3   If you suspect your baby has reflux, even before you get a diagnosis invest in a breathing and movement monitor.

4   Don't try too many different things at once. Try one thing at a time to see what helps and what doesn't.

5   Never try to force your baby to take his milk. There is a very fine line between encouraging him to take enough feed and constantly pushing in that extra ounce, which may cause him to end up with a complete aversion to milk.

6   When introducing a new formula or medication, always give it time to take effect and don't give up on it after just a day or two.

7   Always ask for a second opinion or to be referred to another doctor or paediatrician if you are not happy with the advice or diagnosis (or the lack of) from your current medical professional.

☆ *Alison's Golden Rules* ☆

8   It is good to do some of your own research about reflux, but don't be too hasty to think that any general advice you find will help to resolve the issues for your individual baby.

9   Remember, nothing is a 'miracle cure'. Once medication is in place it may still take time for your baby to forget the association between pain and drinking milk. You may also need to adjust his feeding routine and implement sleep-training to bring things finally to a more manageable level.

10   Remember – dealing with a reflux baby is a complete rollercoaster that can cause a ripple-effect of deeply emotional and worrying times through your whole family. Finding the right course of milk, medication and management is the way to the light at the end of the tunnel – and it is there, I promise!

Your Journal

As mentioned throughout this book, it can be very useful to keep a daily record of your baby's feeding pattern and sleep times.

The following pages contain a few blank charts that you can fill in to commence your journal. If you wish to continue it after completing all the charts provided here, then you can devise your own charts either on a computer or just by drawing up some charts by hand in a blank book.

If you ever need to give medication to your baby, then it is a good idea to keep a record of the time and dose that you give and you can record this in the 'comments' column of the chart. However, if you have a baby who has reflux, for instance, and you are giving medicines more than once a day, it would be a good idea to draw up your own charts and include a 'medicine column' where you can properly record the time and doses given each day.

The following are examples and explanations of the terms and abbreviations that you can adapt for your use when filling in your charts. The first line is filled in with an example. There is a further example of a chart in Chapter 4.

B = breast
L = left
R = right
EBM = expressed breast milk
F= formula
W = wet nappy
D = dirty nappy
Meds = medication

Your Journal

Date/day Feed start-time	Breast/side/ duration Bottle/ amount	Nappy	Sleep time from and to	Comment
Tues 12th/ 10am	B. L 40/R 20	W/D	11.15am to 12.30pm	Good feed and settled well for sleep.

Your Journal

Date/day Feed start-time	Breast/side/ duration Bottle/ amount	Nappy	Sleep time from and to	Comment

Your Sleep Diary

As described in detail in Chapter 6, it can be very useful to keep a sleep diary of your baby or child's sleep patterns before starting and while implementing the reassurance sleep-training technique. As with the previous charts for a daily journal, these are provided for you to start keeping a log of your baby's sleep patterns. Alternatively, you can devise your own.

These charts can be as simple or as detailed as you like. Some parents prefer to keep them quite simple and just record the time of each waking, how long the baby was awake for and when they re-settled to sleep. Others choose to keep a more detailed log and chart all the milk feeds/solid meals along with the time of sleep, duration of sleep, how many times they went in to give a reassurance, etc.

The first line of the following chart is filled in with another example to help guide you. A further example can be found in Chapter 6.

Your Sleep Diary

Date/day	Time of feed	Time of sleep/ comment	Time woke/amount of reassurances/time back to sleep	Total sleep
Tues 12th	11am / 150ml	12.15 put down, took 20 mins to settle, visits 5	Woke 1.15pm, went in 8 times, back asleep by 1.30 & slept till 2.30pm	1 hour 40 mins

Your Sleep Diary

Date/day	Time of feed	Time of sleep/ comment	Time woke/amount of reassurances/time back to sleep	Total sleep

Notes

1. Gerdhart, Sue, *Why Love Matters*, Brunner-Routledge, 2004.

2. Yoo, Seung-Schik, et al., 'A deficit in the ability to form new human memories without sleep', *Nature Neuroscience*, NN Publishing Group, February 2007.

3. Mindell, Jodi, quoted in 'Young Children Don't Sleep Enough', *Web*MD.com/health & parenting news, 2004.

4. Byam-Cook, Clare, *What to Expect When You're Breastfeeding – And What If You Can't?* Workman Publishing, 2006.

5. Kramer, Professor Michael, 'The benefits of breastfeeding being over-sold by the NHS', *The Times*, July 2009.

6. Sprott, Jim, *The Cot Death Cover-up?*, Penguin, 1997.

7. Babcock, Debra, quoted in 'Young Children Don't Sleep Enough', *Web*MD.com/health & parenting news, 2004

Bibliography

Babcock, Debra, quoted in 'Young Children Don't Sleep Enough', web article on ADHD, WebMD.com/health & parenting news, 2004.

Barker, Robin, *Baby Love*, M. Evans, 2002.

Borgenicht, Louis, *The Baby Owners' Manual*, Quirk Books, 2003.

British Medical Journal, 2001, 322 [7297:1266].

Byam-Cook, Clare, *What to Expect When You're Breastfeeding – and What if You Can't?*, Workman Publishing, 2006.

Cave, Simon, and Fertleman, Dr Caroline, *Your Baby, Week by Week*, Vermilion, 2007.

Charlish, Anne, *How to Beat Anxiety, Stress and Depression*, The Bristol Group Ltd., 2002.

Davenport, Tracy and Mike, *Acid Reflux in Infants and Children*, SportWork, 2007.

Deacon, Caroline, *Breastfeeding for Beginners*, HarperCollins, 2002.

Department of Health, *Birth to Five*, 2007.

Doherty, Karen, and Coleridge, Georgina, *Seven Secrets of Successful Parenting*, Transworld, 2008.

Eisenberg, Arlene, Murkoff, Heidi and Hathaway, Sandee, *What to Expect the First Year*, Simon & Schuster, 2005.

Ferber, Richard, *Solve Your Child's Sleep Problems*, Dorling Kindersley, 2006.

Ford, Gina, *The Contented Little Baby Book*, Vermilion, 1999.

Friedrich, Elizabeth, and Rowland, Cheryl, *The Twins' Handbook*, Robson Books, 1983.

Frost, Jo, *Confident Baby Care*, Orion Books, 2007.

Gerdhardt, Sue, *Why Love Matters*, Brunner-Routledge, 2004.

Gopnik, Alison, Meltzoff, Andrew and Kuhl, Patricia, *How Babies Think*, Phoenix, 2006

Henderson, Angela, *The Good Sleep Guide*, Hawthorn Press, 2003.

Henschel, Dora, and Inch, Sally, *Breastfeeding – a Guide for Midwives*, Butterworth-Heinemann, 1996.

Hogg, Tracy, and Blau, Melinda, *Secrets of the Baby Whisperer*, Vermilion, 2003.

Karp, Harvey, *The Happiest Baby on the Block*, Bantam Books, 2004.

Karitane Mothercraft Society, *The Baby Book*, Doubleday, 1990.

Kircheimer, Sid, Improve-your-sleep.com 2008/2009, WebMD.com/health news, 2004.

Kramer, Professor Michael, 'The benefits of breastfeeding being oversold by the NHS', *The Times*, July 2009.

Leonard, Dr Rosemary, *The Seven Ages of Woman*, Transworld, 2007.

Mackean, D. G., *Human Life*, John Murray, 1998.

Maclean, Roni, and McNeil, Jean, *Life on the Reflux Roller Coaster*, Publish America, 2003.

Mindell, Jodi, quoted in 'Young Children Don't Sleep Enough'. *WebMD/com/health & parenting news*, 2004.

Pantley, Elizabeth, *The No-cry Sleep Solution*, McGraw-Hill, 2002.

Pulsifer-Anderson, Beth, *The Reflux Book*, Intensive Care Parenting, 2007.

Renfrew, Mary, Fisher, Chloe, and Arms, Suzanne, *The New Bestfeeding: Getting Breastfeeding Right for You*, Celestial Arts, 2000.

Sears, Dr William, and Sears, Martha, *Baby Sleep Book*, Thorsons, 2005.

Sprott, Jim, *The Cot Death Cover-up?*, Penguin, 1997.

Sweet, Betty, with Timan, Denise (eds), *Mayes' Midwifery*, Bailliere Tindall, 1997.

Teich, Jessica, and de Bravo, Brandel France, *Trees Make the Best Mobiles*, St Martin's Griffin, 2002.

Waldeburger, Jennifer, and Spirack, Jill, *The Sleepeasy Solution: the Exhausted Parent's Guide to Getting Your Child to Sleep from Birth to Five Years*, Barnes & Noble, 2007.

Yoo, Seung-Schik, et al., 'A deficit in the ability to form new human memories without sleep', *Nature Neuroscience*, NN Publishing Group, February 2007.

Index

Acknowledgements

My love and thanks go to all my family and friends who have helped and supported me throughout the birth of 'my baby' – this book!

To my mum, who is always there for me, no matter what; to my husband Martin, for his never-ending support and tolerance of my work (sorry for never being at home!), to my very special daughter Chelsea, for her unconditional love, friendship, belief and loyalty; to my grandson Cameron, who brings so much joy to our lives and who was good enough (with his mum's permission and cooperation) to allow me to use his first few months of life as a case study in this book; to my sisters, who have supported me through some recent tough times; and to Rosie and the boys – Vinnie and Billy – who have never complained about the little time that I (their grandma, aka Mops) have had to spend with them during the compilation of my book. Also to my son and his family, who although distant are never far from me.

I also offer my wholehearted thanks to all my clients – many of whom have now become very dear friends. Until now, nearly all my work has come to me through word of mouth and I give a huge thank-you to all who continue to promote my work. Many of my clients filled in questionnaires, assisted with surveys, helped with contacts and contracts, and you have all been the inspiration for compiling this book. And let's not forget all your babies and children, who have responded to my routines and sleep-training with such ease – well, OK, some have been a little more challenging along the way!

My deepest thanks go to Dr Muftah Eltumi for his support and belief in my work, for his professional guidance, for writing the foreword to this book, and most of all for his good-humoured friendship.

I would also like to thank all the other health professionals, from paediatricians and GPs to health visitors and cranial osteopaths, both private and NHS, that I have met along the way, and who have taken time to listen to my opinions, accept my level of knowledge within the baby-care field and have offered me their own support, help, advice and views which have been so very helpful.

Last but by no means least, I would like to give my sincerest thanks to all those at Transworld who have helped bring my dream to reality. Special thanks go to my editor Brenda Kimber, for understanding and believing in me at the start and for promoting my project to the rest of the team, which led to the commission of this book. Being a complete novice author and not having anyone as a grand a literary agent, I have valued her guidance on this journey from contract to publication. She has given me masses of help and support and had the patience of a saint. Thank you again to all the team for bringing this book to life – it wouldn't have happened without you!

With wonderful memories of my best friend Fiona, who sits in her poppy field up on high, but is always with me. Thank you xx.

Alison Scott-Wright started her 'caring' career at sixteen in a nursing home for the elderly, and worked in the nursing profession for the next few years. She had two children during her early twenties, so was kept very busy as a working mum. In the early 1990s she set up and ran her own very successful community home-care/nursing agency, at one time employing over thirty staff. It was after this, in 1995, that she took her first position as a maternity nurse, working with a mum and her newborn twins, and finally discovered her real passion in life - babies. Since then she has never looked back.

Alison quickly discovered that she had almost a 'sixth sense' where babies are concerned, and based her career on this intuitive understanding of them. Along the way she has trained in, and researched in depth, various aspects of baby care, as well as basic counselling, communication and listening skills, postnatal depression and family dynamics. Over the years she has learned that babies are relatively easy to understand and manage; adults, however, are much more complex and require a far more sensitive approach!

Alison realized that the common but distressing condition of reflux in babies can cause many more problems than just the odd bit of sick or crying, and that if undiagnosed and untreated, it can result in ongoing sleep problems, long-term negative and unhealthy associations with food, and disturbing behavioural issues as babies move into toddlerhood. This has since become a specialist area in her work and she is continually trying to raise awareness and understanding of reflux in babies. Her other specialist field is sleep – or the lack of it – in babies, and she has been named the 'Magic Sleep Fairy' by many of her clients.

Alison lives in Swanage, Dorset in a very happy household with her husband, daughter, grandson, mother (part-time), two dogs and three cats. She has even taken work home with her on occasion by having babies come and stay, making it almost a family business! By always looking on the positive side, and keeping her sense of humour, she is able to dedicate much of her time to parents and babies who are in need of help.